IVC hub in
St. A. city n
LH side of hospital CP.

Unforgotten

Life Course, Culture and Aging: Global Transformations
General Editor: Jay Sokolovsky, University of South Florida St. Petersburg

Published by Berghahn Books under the auspices of the Association for Anthropology and Gerontology (AAGE) and the American Anthropological Association Interest Group on Aging and the Life Course

The consequences of aging will influence most areas of contemporary life around the globe: the makeup of households and communities; systems of care; generational exchange and kinship; the cultural construction of the life cycle; symbolic representations of midlife, elderhood and old age; and attitudes toward health, disability and life's end. This series will publish monographs and collected works that examine these widespread transformations with a perspective on the entire life course as well as mid/late adulthood, engaging a cross-cultural framework. It will explore the role of older adults in changing cultural spaces and how this evolves in our rapidly globalizing planet.

Volume 1
TRANSITIONS AND TRANSFORMATIONS
Cultural Perspectives on Aging and the Life Course
Edited by Caitrin Lynch & Jason Danely

Volume 2
UNFORGOTTEN
Love and the Culture of Dementia Care in India
Bianca Brijnath

Titles in Preparation:

AGEING AND THE DIGITAL LIFE COURSE
Edited by David Prendergast & Chiara Garattini

WALTZING INTO OLD AGE
Redefining Aging, the Life Course and Eldercare in China
Hong Zhang

UNFORGOTTEN

Love and the Culture of Dementia Care in India

By

Bianca Brijnath

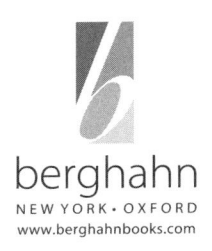

berghahn
NEW YORK · OXFORD
www.berghahnbooks.com

Published in 2014 by
Berghahn Books
www.berghahnbooks.com

© 2014 Bianca Brijnath

All rights reserved.
Except for the quotation of short passages for the purposes
of criticism and review, no part of this book may be reproduced
in any form or by any means, electronic or mechanical,
including photocopying, recording, or any information
storage and retrieval system now known or to be invented,
without written permission of the publisher.

Library of Congress Cataloging-in-Publication Data

Brijnath, Bianca.
 Unforgotten: love and the culture of dementia care in India / by Bianca Brijnath.
  pages cm -- (Life course, culture and aging: global transformations; volume 2)
 Includes bibliographical references and index.
  ISBN 978-1-78238-354-3 (hardback: alk. paper) -- ISBN 978-1-78238-355-0 (ebook)
  1. Senile dementia--Patients--Care--India. 2. Senile dementia--Patients--Family relationships--India. 3. Caregivers--India. I. Title.
  RC524.B75 2014
  616.8'300954--dc23

2014016236

British Library Cataloguing in Publication Data
A catalogue record for this book is
available from the British Library.

ISBN 978-1-78238-354-3 (hardback)
ISBN 978-1-78238-355-0 (ebook)

For my grandparents, Hazel and Dara Balsara

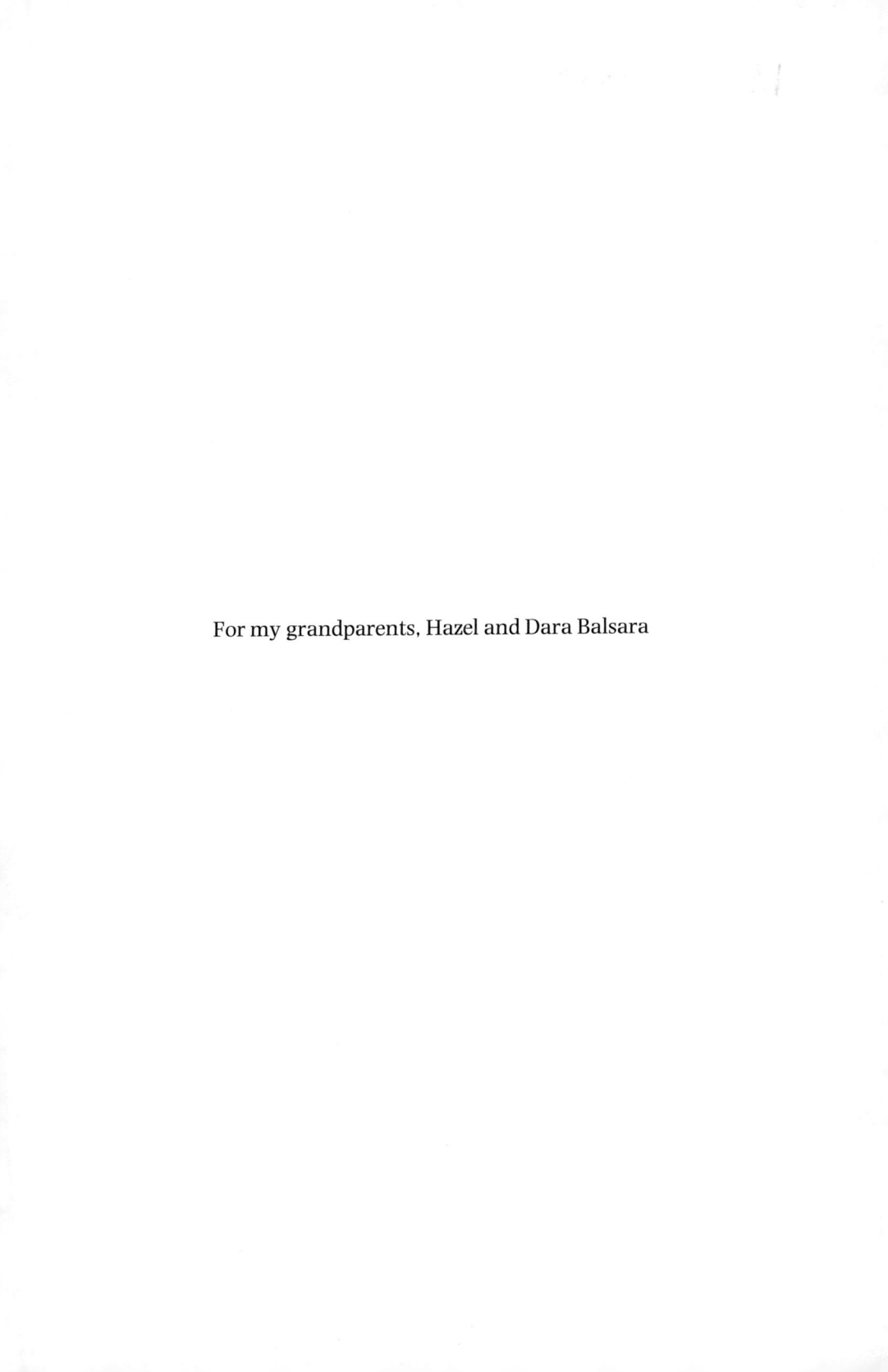

🖎 = context

CONTENTS

List of Illustrations — viii
Acknowledgements — ix
Notes on Transliteration — xi

Introduction — 1
Chapter 1. Methods and Character Building — 12
Chapter 2. The Diagnostic Process — 38
Chapter 3. Therapeutics and Health Seeking — 59
Chapter 4. The Economies of Care — 87
Chapter 5. Alzheimer's and the Indian Appetite — 116
Chapter 6. Stigma and Loneliness in Care — 137
Chapter 7. The Journey to Silence — 157
Conclusion. 'This is the Time for Romance' — 183

Glossary — 192
References — 194
Index — 217

ILLUSTRATIONS

Figures

Figure 1.1	The silk-cotton tree outside my *barsathi*	18
Figure 1.2	Delhi on the move	19
Figure 1.3	ARDSI volunteers training poor women to be home attendants	22
Figure 3.1	Concurrent use of biomedical *ilāj* by people living with dementia	72
Figure 4.1	Kamini's women, training to be paid attendants	109
Figure 5.1	Shivbaksh Chand cooking	124
Figure 7.1	An afternoon shave	166
Figure 7.2	An afternoon nap	170
Figure 7.3	Beautiful Gauri	170
Figure 7.4	Playing carom	171
Figure 7.5	Men at work	171
Figure 7.6	Helen Meena Chand, 1926–2008	177

Tables

Table 1.1	Demographic data of families	25
Table 4.1	Costs of care for a person with dementia	91
Table 7.1	Comparing cultural scripts on dying in Anglophone and Asian countries	175

ACKNOWLEDGEMENTS

THIS BOOK IS THE PRODUCT of many peoples' labour and therefore there are many who must be acknowledged. First and foremost I thank Lenore Manderson for her generosity of spirit and intellect; I was privileged to have been her student.

I also thank my compatriots when I was at the Social Science and Health Research Unit at Monash University; Ajay Ranjan Singh, Surekha Garimella, Shyamala Nataraj and Narelle Warren were generous in their time and willingness to develop ideas with me. I am also most grateful to Arthur Kleinman, Annemarie Mol and Sarah Lamb for reading drafts of various chapters. Their comments, encouragement and recommendations for further reading have significantly strengthened the analysis. Lawrence Cohen and Annette Leibing examined this work in its doctoral format; their comments and criticisms have been incorporated into this manuscript and have significantly strengthened it. The comments of two anonymous reviewers further tightened the analysis as did the gentle prompting of my series editor, Jay Sokolovsky, to incorporate more cross-cultural dimensions into the work. Ann Przyzycki DeVita, Molly Mosher, Charlotte Mosedale and Ben Parker from Berghahn Books were swift to respond to my queries and guide me through the publication process.

Alzheimer's Australia, the Australian Federal Government and Monash University financially supported the initial fieldwork and PhD through an Alzheimer's Australia Postgraduate Scholarship for Social Research in Dementia (2010–2009), the Endeavour Research Fellowship (2008) and a Monash University Graduate Scholarship (2008–2007). The Australian National Health and Medical Research Council gave me the room to finalize this manuscript through their postdoctoral fellowship programme. I am deeply grateful for all this support.

Without the aid of the Alzheimer's and Related Disorders Society of India (ARDSI) this project would not have been possible. I thank Dr Jacob Roy, Mrs Nirmala Narula, Colonel Khanna, Veena Sachdeva, Y.P. Singh, Renu Vohra, Ranita Ray and Vijay Seth. I am in awe of their dedication; most work on a voluntary basis and juggle a hundred other commitments. My faith in ARDSI's capacity to achieve great things is increasingly borne out by their successes – there is now a day-care centre in Delhi offering short-term respite care to families caring for a loved one with dementia.

During my fieldwork in India, I received understated yet terrific guidance from Dr Deepak Mehta and a home and hot food from Sanjay Srivastava and Radha Khan during the cold early days in Delhi. Param and Bhagirathi Saikia, Aditya Sikand and Rajen and Roma Brijnath provided havens when I needed them. Harinder Baweja, Kavita Muthana, Archana Mahapatra, Nupur Maskara, Sunena Jain and Namita Bhandare aided me in various ways from curtains to coffees to *kadhi* – I thank you.

My family – David Tittensor, Rohit and Sarah Brijnath, the Balsara and Brijnath clans – accepted my shortage of time, temper and grace yet still encouraged me to persevere. I thank my aunt Kumud Sikand for allowing me to use her painting 'Alzheimer's' for the cover of this book and David McMahon for photographing this artwork. Most especially, I thank my husband David for his critical commentary, his willingness to engage, his brutal honesty on my drafts and for giving me the final, ignominious push to stop procrastinating and publish this book.

Last but not least, to the carers and families who shared their stories with me – words cannot express how much I appreciate and value this gift of intimacy. These narratives are carried in my head and my heart. I hope that I have done them justice in the following pages.

NOTES ON TRANSLITERATION

ALL HINDI WORDS ARE ITALICIZED. I used the Digital Dictionaries of South Asia (see http://dsal.uchicago.edu/dictionaries/about.html) for the spelling and diacritics of Hindi words in English. Specifically, I relied on Mahendra Caturvedi's *A Practical English-Hindi Dictionary* and John T. Platt's *A Dictionary of Urdu, Classical Hindi, and English*. To be consistent with the dictionary spellings, a few words have not been spelt as they are popularly used (e.g., *cha:y* instead of *chai*). Where I have not been able to locate the word in the dictionaries (e.g., *barsathi*), I have used my own spelling without diacritics. Only film and book titles are cited as in the original.

When Hindi words first appear they are translated. If the word is only used once and adequately explained in the text, I have excluded it from the glossary for brevity. Hindi sentences and/or colloquial mixtures of Hindi and English are accompanied by English translations in parentheses. Brackets have only been used to either clarify the speaker's meaning or to illustrate the tone of the speech. All my dialogue is italicized to distinguish it from my participants' speech. All translations of interviews from Hindi to English have been undertaken by me and I alone am responsible for any errors.

INTRODUCTION

Dear Grandma,
I will always remember you, especially your hands. The hands that made us pish-pash and doused it in ketchup. The hands that hid forgotten treasures in your cupboard, kept under lock and key. The hands that gestured so wildly when you told me stories about how naughty Des used to be. The hands that bathed me and covered me head-to-toe in talcum powder. They have always been the softest hands. I always felt very special when I was with you. I will never forget the kind of love that you showed me and all your grandchildren. We were all truly privileged to have a Grandma like you.
I will always love you.

My grandmother Hazel died on 4 March 2012. These heartfelt words are from my cousin's note that was read at her funeral and slipped into her casket. Arriving at this sad and solemn moment was a long journey for my family, one that has extended well over a decade. We observed the loss of a woman – physically, mentally and relationally – and with each loss, my grandmother has demanded from us an explicit acknowledgement of what it means to care. Her every deterioration, the pneumonia, the fractured hip, the infected gums, the shuttered eyes, exacted a toll. But we were not the victims of her dementia, merely the witnesses to it. It was our job to see her pain and suffering, pay her hospital and medical bills, endure the familial and marital strains created by her illness, cancel holidays and eventually plan her funeral. Now that she is gone, we are charged with the responsibilities of remembering her and remembering what we saw.

To care for someone with dementia[1] is no easy task. It requires confrontation with your own humanity and your limitations. You are sometimes unrecognizable in your capacity for tenderness, for the depths of your cruelty. I never imagined I would derive so much pleasure from feeding my grandmother. I never imagined I would experience such rage when I overfed her and had to clean her diarrhoea nine times in two days. None of us ever imagined we could be our grandmother's doctor, nurse, beautician, intimate cleaner, teacher, disciplinarian and historian, charged with the dual tasks of caring for and about (Lynch and McLaughlin 1995). But in taking on these roles, our family irrevocably changed. I have irrevocably changed.

This book is about such transformative practices, about immutable change through care, the *joie de vivre* of the care relationship, its shadows and eventual death. It is about how middle-class families in urban Delhi look after a loved one with dementia; about how people of means and education, in a globalized, urbanized and ageing world, grapple with the personal experience of caregiving, the functioning of stigma in daily life, the social and cultural barriers in accessing support and the meanings invested in these processes. It is about how spouses such as Shivbaksh Chand, Nina Bhagat, Govind Ballabh Tandon and Josie Dharam Singh[2] reordered their moral and social worlds, changed traditional gender roles and struggled to retain a relationship in the face of disruption and change; about how children like Namita Sood, Nayantara Sen and Suneeta Sadhwani took on parental roles and dealt with the rancour of attendants, family politics and community perceptions. The analyses presented in this book will speak to the complexities of care, ageing, culture and love within families in an era of modernity, money and socio-economic change. Simultaneously it shows how cultural frameworks historically specific to India, such as medical pluralism and hope for a cure, the emotional currency of feeding and eating and the powerful bonds of kinship and reciprocity, continue to structure everyday worlds and practices.

Why Dementia, Why India, Why Now?

Since Lawrence Cohen's (1998) exemplary book *No Aging in India*, there has been no further ethnographic work in India that has focused on the experiences of age-related dementia care. This is quite remarkable as the subject of ageing and all that is associated with it is a conversation that needs to be had in India, particularly in light of the rapid socio-economic and demographic changes that are taking place. As a result of these changes there are many pressing questions that need to be answered. Namely, what will happen in 2030 when nineteen per cent of the Indian population, about 300 million people, are over sixty years old (WHO 2012)? How can Indian families and the formal health and care systems prepare when the projected 346 per cent increase in dementia prevalence occurs by 2040 (Ferri et al. 2005)? These are some of the very real and serious challenges that Indian society will have to confront in the not-too-distant future. As such, the narratives presented here offer some insight into what is to come.

It is imperative that we start to engage with and answer these questions. For, while the current standard prevalence rates for dementia are low, ranging between 8.2 per cent for urban Indian settings and 8.7 per cent for rural Indian settings (Rodriguez et al.. 2008), the actual numbers of people living with dementia are relatively high. In 2001, 1.5 million Indians were estimated to have dementia, the third highest number in the world (Ferri et al. 2005); in 2010, 3.7 million Indians were estimated to have dementia (ARDSI 2010). Though no reliable data is available for Delhi, where my research was conducted in 2008, the Alzheimer's and Related Disorders Society of India – Delhi Chapter estimated that approximately 15,000 people were living with dementia at that time. Through undertaking research into dementia care in India we can be anticipatory in addressing systemic shortages and implementing culturally appropriate care arrangements. More importantly we can gain a deeper understanding of the cross-cutting and culturally specific meanings associated with ageing, care and reason, in the face of such profound degeneration and loss.

Meanings of Dementia: Cross-Cultural Perspectives

Research has consistently shown, in India, that dementia and its primary symptom 'memory loss' have been perceived as a normal part of ageing (see Emmatty, Bhatti and Mukalel 2006; Patel and Prince 2001; Shaji et al. 2002; Trivedi 2003). *Saṭhiyānā* or 'gone sixtyish', in north Indian local vernacular, was identified by Lawrence Cohen (1998) in the 1990s as broadly describing the mental symptoms of dementia – memory loss (*bhūlnā*), stubbornness (*ẓid*), increased aggression (*guṣṣa*), paranoia and suspicion.[3] Similar conceptions exist in other parts of India: *chinnan* ('childishness') in Malayalam (Iype et al. 2006) and *nerva frakese* ('tired brain') in Konkani (Patel and Prince 2001).

Work undertaken elsewhere in Asia has also identified local idioms associated with dementia and ageing (see Ikels 2002; Traphagan 2009). Rather than being a mere change in terminology, these linguistic differences also signal variations in understandings and symptoms of dementia and more broadly about health. In China, mental function is not equated with cognitive capacity, for as long as a person is doing what is right in terms of the observance of social roles, he/she is seen to be thinking 'rationally' with both heart and mind (Ikels 2002). In Japan, *boke* or senility is not seen as a disease but as a condition preventable through being physically and mentally active and socially engaged (Traphagan 1998).

These local idioms of dementia not only reflect how understandings of illness are rooted in social rather than medical pathology but also that there are gaps in the public health system when it comes to raising awareness and facilitating early diagnosis and management. In India, for example, there is little awareness in the medical fraternity, excepting specialists such as neurologists and psychiatrists, about how to diagnose and treat people living with dementia. This is due to the very limited inclusion of dementia in medical curriculum (although this is changing) and the acute shortage of mental health professionals (0.3 psychiatrists and 0.03 social workers per 100,000 population) (WHO 2011). Combined with poor infrastructure, inadequate supply of drugs, too few trained staff and the use of culturally-inappropriate treatment models, as well as patient barriers that are either self-imposed or generated within the family or by its circumstances, it comes as little surprise that dementia may be regarded as a social phenomenon, clinically under-diagnosed and poorly managed (Gururaj, Girish and Issac 2005; Thara, Padmavati and Srinivasan 2004).

When compared to Western concepts of dementia the differences are stark. Memory loss, functional decline and cognitive impairment are associated with a loss of personhood, dignity and quality of life. Sharon Kaufman (2006: 23) describes the construction of dementia in the West as 'a condition both of death-in-life and of life-in-death'. The risk of dementia or even a potential diagnosis of mild cognitive impairment is often met with such fear and anxiety that some individuals delay contacting a health professional about their memory problems (Corner and Bond 2004, 2006; Townsend, Godfrey and Denby 2006). While there is tacit acknowledgement that with ageing comes a decline in physical and mental health, in the West, people with dementia are often viewed as pitiful, dependent and without a sense of self (Ballenger 2006; Townsend et al. 2006). Although efforts have been made to change this perception, within the wider context of ageing, infirmity and self-management, the image of the ageing dementing person remains a source of considerable anxiety and fear in Western settings (Ballenger 2006).

This brief comparison of the multiple meanings of dementia cross-culturally highlights that old age, like middle age, youth or childhood, is never just a chronological and biological marker of the life process, but also reflects culturally specific values, beliefs and practices determining the behaviour of people among and towards the old. Meanings and presentations of dementia vary by culture, language, income, education, conflicting beliefs about health and thus also determine patterns of health-seeking and its management (Cohen 2006). By recognizing how in some cultures, bodily decline and degeneration, which require medical intervention can co-exist alongside 'normal' ageing, which allows for physical and mental infirmities and dysfunctions requiring familial and not medical care, different narratives of care emerge and insight is provided into how some cultures appropriate dementia care into existing care frameworks.

Traditional Forms of Elder Care in India

Traditionally, like other forms of care in India, elder care was organized under the joint family system. Parents, children and grandchildren all lived in the same house, theoretically (if not always literally) sharing property and income. The familial structure was patriarchal – men controlled social and economic matters, women managed household and other general affairs (Bhat and Dhruvarajan 2001; Prakash 1999).

According to Vedic Hindu philosophy, a person's life was demarcated into four life-stages or *ashramas*, through which the person was meant to progress: *brahmacharya* (studentship and learning), *grahasthya* (married householder), *vanaprastha* (a disengaged forest dweller) and *sanyas* (a wandering ascetic) (Kane 1930, 1962; The Laws of Manu c. 500 BC). The last two phases, which denote the process of disengagement from the minutiae of everyday life and deeper introspection of a more metaphysical sort, rarely occur in practice (Rao 1993). Instead older people continue to live with their children and remain involved in their lives and there is a social expectation of care from their children based on intergenerational reciprocation and the importance of doing *sevā* (Lamb 2000; Vatuk 1990).

Sevā, literally service, is a layered concept that links the social body to individual ones. It is the intellectual, emotional and physical care of elders based on respect, with such care likened to a form of divine worship (Vatuk 1990). In the act of seeking *pra-ṇām* (blessing), for example, a younger person bends down to touch the dust of an older person's feet to their head, exactly as devotees do to the figures of their deities (Lamb 2000). Older people are revered and younger people are expected to comply with their requests, seek their advice and follow it, not argue or talk back and display appropriate respect by always using familial titles to address them (*dādā* – paternal grandfather; *dādī* – paternal grandmother) or the more generic 'uncle' and 'aunty' for unrelated elders (Lamb 2000). There are also more tactile dimensions to *sevā*. Younger people, most often the *bahūs* (daughters-in-law), are expected to serve older family members their meals, indulge them with treats (usually sweets), launder and mend their clothes and lay their bedding. More physical, intimate aspects of care such as massaging legs, oiling backs, combing and braiding hair and even bathing and toileting infirm elders are also performed as a part of *sevā* (Lamb 2000).

Sevā is not a simple hierarchical relationship whereby younger people are subjugated and older people deified. To provide *sevā* is also to exercise power, to reveal the decline and decay of ageing bodies and symbolically to relocate older people to the peripheries of everyday domesticity (Cohen 1998; Lamb 2000). The social expectations of performing *sevā*, the acts mandated by it – feeding, cleaning, clothing, sheltering, listening – underlie the disciplinary transitions that ageing bodies and ageing identities must undergo: from doing to accepting; from authoritative to ethereal selves. Similarly, *sevā* serves to discipline younger family members, to set out the types of activities they should perform and where they should perform them.

Dementia disrupts this traditional power dynamic. The loss of memory, the loss of the ability to give *pra-ṇām*, the loss of continence and the loss of ability to care for oneself, irrespective of whether the older person ever formally cared for themselves, shift the perception of ageing bodies from wise to worn out. This is reflected in local languages used to describe dementia (e.g., tired brain, gone sixtyish). Also there are cognitive assumptions that underpin *sevā*. Sylvia Vatuk's (1990) work on ageing in Delhi found that while older people felt they had a legitimate right to be supported and cared for by their adult children, they simultaneously experienced a kind of 'dependency anxiety' that they would be a burden upon the finances, labour and emotional resources of the household. This dependency anxiety only applied in circumstances where the older person felt that their physical or mental health was deteriorating. If that were to occur, then they felt that their position within the family would alter from being in receipt of *sevā* to being dependent or subordinate to their children, i.e., moving from the role of venerated elder to that of needy person (Vatuk 1990). These traditional notions of *sevā* and how dementia disrupts the ageing dyads of young/old, energetic/passive, deference/advisory is a key theme that will be explored throughout the course of this book.

The Wicked Spectre of Modernity

Adding a further layer of complexity is the fact that traditional paradigms of care have been and continue to be transformed by 'modernity', i.e. forces such as globalization, migration, urbanization, consumerism and the changing role of women. Migration, whether from rural villages to urban cities or from India to overseas, is changing familial structures with older family members sometimes being left behind. In parts of India this has given rise to a common acronym – PICA – Parents in India, Children Abroad (Prince and Trebilco 2005). Women's roles in India have also changed from that of home-based primary carer to full-time paid worker, even after marriage. Consequently women have a reduced availability and willingness to care and families overall are less likely to be able to meet all the medical, social, financial and psychological needs of older family members (Patel and Prince 2001).

When combined with urbanization, growth in consumerism and the adoption of supposedly more 'Western lifestyles', there is a perception that older people are not as securely positioned in their family hierarchy nor are they as revered as was the case in previous generations (Dharmalingam 1994; Jamuna 2003; Kumar 1996; Mahajan 2006). The venerated role of the older person in society is assumed to have diminished, thereby resulting in their increasing maltreatment, loneliness and poor state of health.

This 'wicked spectre' of modernity is far-reaching and powerful. Both Cohen (1998) and Lamb (2000) found a link in popular discourse and in Indians' perceptions of a 'bad' old age and modernity. In Cohen's (1998: 17) comprehensive analysis of Indian gerontology, he notes that when the 'universalist' biomedical languages of dementia are interpreted through cultural and moral filters, dementia is not just plaques and tangles in brains but also a 'senile pathology . . . located in family dynamics and cultural crisis'. Modernity creates 'bad' fractured families where a lack of respect for the aged translates into greater numbers of older people being senile and demented.

Similarly Sarah Lamb (2009) in her work on old age homes in Kolkata canvassed the vehement positive and negative public reactions to these sites, concluding that Indians take such emerging and novel modes of serving the ageing to '[r]epresent a profound transformation – a transformation involving not only ageing per se, but principles underlying the very foundation of society and the identity of India as a nation and culture' (Lamb 2009: 89).

This inverse relation between modernity and ageing has also been observed in other parts of the world (for reviews see Aboderin 2004; Holmes and Holmes 1995). However, it has come under sharp criticism from different quarters with research from Europe (Savla et al. 2008), Australia (Baldassar, Baldock and Wilding 2007), China (Zhang 2009) and Mexico (Sokolovsky 2009a) showing that far from only creating hardship for older people, modernity has also been beneficial and has wrought new ways of being in families. Sokolovsky (2009b: 179) has argued that 'Global transformations are not necessarily a horrible thing for the aged if their locality has some control over key resources and older citizens are included in the process of figuring out what adaptations are best for the community'.

Echoing Sokolovsky's point, Lamb (2009) also observed in her later study that while the wicked spectre of modernity continued to loom over the gerontological and media landscape in India, its shadow had diminished and that in actual practice older people and their carers enunciated far more ambiguous and complex understandings of ageing and care.

This is a remarkable and substantive change since the earlier writings of Cohen (1998) and Lamb (2000). In just over a decade perceptions have shifted in India, absorbing the language of globalization, biomedicine and modernity, appropriating and indigenizing concepts in different ways, forging more nuanced and less oppositional understandings of modernity, ageing, illness and care. Notably, I found in Delhi that the term *saṭhiyānā* that Cohen (1998) reported as characterizing so much of his interlocutors' perceptions of dementia was hardly mentioned. There are numerous explanations for the lack of use of this term,[4] including the fact that many of the families I worked with were 'medicalized' through the diagnostic process, which had replaced their language of senility and a normal old age with a language of illness and care. However, the wider absence of the term *saṭhiyānā* in everyday parlance also signals a major shift in the iteration of dementia in India's urban middle class. Take for example this computer-savvy carer's explanation for how he understood dementia:

> It is like an XP® operating system and you have Microsoft Office®. The operating system is separate and then you add whatever is in your biochemical environment interactions or interface. As you grow old, these things you lose but the basic operating system remains the same. The operating system is given in everybody, but what you have learned in your life and what I have learned in my life is different and this is the only thing that is lost in dementia or in Alzheimer's as you call it.

In this carer's words, we hear an understanding of dementia as being rooted in technology, class and age, rather than the perils of modernity and 'bad' families. The cultural specificity of a middle-class, middle-aged well educated Delhi-ite is heard in this carer's voice, but so too is an understanding of illness that is identifiable to those even with minimal technical know-how across the world. The stamp of capitalism and Microsoft's monopoly is felt, as well as the effects of technology on everyday life. Dementia, as articulated by this carer, is a dialogic product of medicine, culture and technology. Modernity is no longer just the 'wicked spectre', rather it can now also provide an alternate framework to explain the relationship between age and dementia.

Towards an Anthropology of Dementia Care

To date much of the writings on age and dementia care have come from the disciplines of nursing, sociology and gerontology. Nursing has tended to examine 'bath and body work' and the skill sets required to complete these tasks (Foner 1994; Lee-Treweek 1997; Schumacher et al. 2000; Twigg 2000). Both sociology and women's studies tend to explore the emotional labour invested in carework, especially as a private feminized form of unpaid, unvalued labour (Askham et al. 2007; Hibberd et al. 2009; Hochschild 1989; Moe 2003; Victor et al. 2000), while gerontology has focused on the impact of caregiving on carers, the coping mechanisms and the support systems needed (Brodaty and Green 2002; Ory et al. 1999; Schulz and Martire 2004; Vitaliano, Zhang and Scanlan 2003). The language of 'perceived burden', 'psychosocial stress' and 'coping mediators' can sometimes characterize these literatures with the result that the emotional and physical work of care is obfuscated and the moral and affective dimensions unaddressed.

Recent anthropological writings have made significant inroads in this regard by examining the meanings and textures of care. Contributions from Arthur Kleinman (2008, 2009), Janelle Taylor (2008), Pia Kontos (2006, 2007) and Annette Leibing (2002, 2006) have illustrated that care comprises a complex, layered set of practices embedded in relations of power, pathos, identity and morality. Kleinman (2009: 293) who cared for his wife, Joan, who had dementia, captures it eloquently:

> Caregiving is also a defining moral practice. It is a practice of empathic imagination, responsibility, witnessing and solidarity with those in great need. It is a moral practice that makes caregivers, and at times even the care-receivers, more present and thereby fully human.

Similarly, Mol (2008: 1) makes the point that carework encompasses tasks that 'make daily life more bearable'. Carework is not about achieving a cure, though it may sometimes lead to one, but about an ethical engagement, a process of meaning-making and sometimes even re-making people, about reminding and remembering people for who they were and finding the pleasures and relationality in who they are (Taylor 2008). It is about identifying what really matters in the care relationship.

In this book, I am explicitly concerned with the transformative processes that illness and degeneration create and how this transformation occurs in contemporary urban India, which has undergone substantial economic, social and material changes in the last decade. I will argue that what really characterizes the dementia care relationship is love and transformation, something that has hitherto not been explored in the familial setting in contemporary urban India. From the husband who wakes up at 3 A.M. to feed ice-cream to his wife with late-stage dementia because that is the time when she is most responsive, the wife who refuses to admit that her husband will not get better because that would mean giving up on him and accepting he will die and the two daughters who gave up work for seven years and spent all their resources to care for their ageing mother with dementia, because that is what caring means to them, there is an enormous amount of drama, pathos and tragedy in the care relationship and the meanings in these activities need to be unravelled.

Book Overview

To begin I outline the methods that underpin this study. I then take the reader on a spatial journey that starts in the home, moves to the hospital and back again (Chapters 2, 3 and 4). In Chapter 2 the heuristic processes of diagnosis, of 'seeing', 'showing' and 'being seen', are discussed. I argue that diagnosis is not a straight-forward process but occurs with time and in stages. In describing this diagnostic journey I will show how the diagnosis marks the beginning of a road of caring for a person living with dementia. In Chapter 3 various practices, such as doctor shopping, are contextualized via an analysis of the history of the doctor-patient relationship in India and multiple meanings of health are explored. In particular, I focus on how power and medicine are intertwined, on the effects of medications and on the hope that people seek from a cure. In Chapter 4, I explore the costs people incur in carework, the subjective emotional hurts they bear and the objective financial outlays they expend. In these chapters, I also describe the environments that care is given in, the resource scarcities of the public health system, the pressures doctors work under, the exploitations by class and the agency of people in this terrain.

In Chapters 5, 6 and 7, I move away from the medical to explicate social and cultural aspects of care. In Chapter 5, I examine the critical role of food – cooking, feeding and eating – in carework. Food and its links to *sevā*, citizenship, hunger, waste and love are examined, as is the role of surveillance and management of the body. In Chapter 6, I build on the theme of surveillance by unpacking how the bodies of people with dementia are managed to mitigate stigma. I question whether there is a stigma attached to people with dementia and return to the heuristic processes of 'seeing', discussed in Chapter 2. But here I show that the gaze is inverted as one is asked to see normality in abnormality. Stigma, I argue, need not be dramatic and deep to be grievous. Rather, it may happen through small slights that, when combined, create feelings of pain and isolation.

Chapter 7 uses the elements of a Bollywood film to listen to the voices of people with dementia. I illustrate that through song, dance and poetry, relationships can be formed and people may express themselves in creative and poignant ways. I also explore death and dying in dementia, describing how people conceive of death, the political economy of dying and the new biopolitics of capitalism and organ donation.

Lastly, I explore the theme of love. Love flows implicitly throughout this work, both in the intimacies that people with dementia and their families share with each other and in the love I feel for this work. This has been the happiest discovery of my intellectual journey: the personal and professional intimacies that I have been privy to and have tried to express. I acknowledge that my feelings may bias my analysis; however, I also think they attune me to the moral and ethical imperatives in care thus yielding a richer analysis.

Notes

1. I follow the linguistic practices of my interlocutors in interchangeably using the terms dementia and Alzheimer's. I acknowledge that the term 'dementia' has been recently replaced in the clinical language by the term 'major neurocognitive disorder' (The American Psychiatric Association 2013) but I have chosen not to use the latter term because it is clunky, awkward and would be unfamiliar to the families that participated in my study.
2. Pseudonyms have been used for all participants mentioned in this book.
3. There is no specific word for paranoia or suspicion in everyday Hindi. It is explained via an analogy or through direct example.
4. Causes for this research discrepancy may include location (Cohen's work was largely based in Varanasi, mine in Delhi), local cultures (Varanasi is a religious centre for Hindus, Delhi the political capital of India), changes over time in people's attitudes (from the early 1990s to 2008) and different research cohorts (Cohen's work focused on understanding meanings of senility, age and madness amongst a cross-section of Indian society whereas mine concentrated principally on middle-class and elite families).

1. METHODS AND CHARACTER BUILDING

I KEPT DIARIES FROM 1 January 2008 to 10 October 2008. Volumes were filled in coffee shops, temples, stairwells and at my desk, on my fieldwork experiences, frustrations and longings for Australia and my de facto partner, who was on his own fieldwork adventure elsewhere. These journals gave me great comfort, offering an avenue to vent and tangible evidence of my efforts at gathering data. I am deeply attached to them. To my mind they signal my anthropological rite of passage and offer an insight into the messiness of my personal growth. I see in these diaries honest descriptors of what Nita Kumar (1992: 1) defines as fieldwork, 'that brash, awkward, hit-and-run encounter of one sensibility with others'.

I draw on these diaries to contextualize my experiences and explain the methods used to collect data. While on the one hand, I recount a rigorous, evidence-based approach, I balance this against the specificities of India and the habitus of my participants' lives. The research design, participant recruitment, interviews and observations, techniques of analysis and limitations of the study will be outlined, alongside the cultural idiosyncrasies of my interviews. My participants often perceived me as a doctor, interrupted interviews, displayed consent in unique ways and confounded any attempts to categorize them. I return to these themes later.

For me, fieldwork was an intensely personal experience where few things were done purely for scientific reasons. Such an observation could apply to most research projects, shaped as they are by the serendipitous unfolding of funding priorities, ethics committees, fieldwork demands and the researcher's own biases in analyses and written representations. These hidden subjectivities and more obvious drivers often create discrepancies between what is outlined on paper and what was enacted in practice. The methods initially proposed may differ significantly from what was done and there can be solid justifications for such changes – cultural differences in conceiving researcher-participant relations, inappropriateness of certain scales and questionnaires to particular contexts and hitherto unexplored avenues that are only discovered once in the field, which merit further investigation. Additionally in-situ gender, class and race relations, language proficiencies and wider forces of globalization, capital and politics determine whether methods need to be changed. Such points are not new and are well documented in anthropological journals and methods textbooks.

But in illustrating the discrepancies between methods-on-paper and methods-in-practice, there is a risk of compromising the 'scientific' validity of the work and leaving one's credibility open to question. Should an early career researcher write about ruptures in her methods in her first book? I draw counsel from my anthropological elder Paul Rabinow (1977: 5) who argues that if the strengths of anthropology lie in its experiential, reflective and critical capacities, then it behoves anthropologists to challenge the positivism of those projects that aim to study human behaviours without accounting for their own humanities.

Research Design

This study used a critical and sensory ethnographic approach to explore the lived experiences of families caring for people with dementia in India. Critical ethnography incorporates observation and interviews and a dialectic relationship with the discipline of anthropology itself. The focus is on relationships, language and objects of encounter in local and transnational settings, flows of power, the effects of political and economic forces alongside culture, the reflexivity of the ethnographer to these factors and their own subjectivity and influence on the research (Herzfeld 1987; Marcus 1995).

By marrying this approach to a sensorial anthropology (Nichter 2008; Pink 2009), I have examined the way in which these foci are experienced and responded to sensorially (touch, taste, smell, sounds) and the positive and negative connotations imbued within these experiences. How, for example, are sensory markers of dementia care – such as incontinence, violence and feeding – experienced and perceived within middle-class Indian families? What trade-offs occur between carers and their wider social environ when the former undertake interpersonal and intrapersonal care for a person with dementia? Can 'real' kin, distanced and far away, be replaced by 'fictive' kin, immediate and tactile?

These were the questions that I was concerned with in my data collection and analysis. My aim was to try to capture people's worlds and the structures that underpin them. Reliability and validity were ensured by the triangulation of interview (n=74) and observational data (approximately 250 hours), discourse analysis and document reviews (Angen 2000; Whittemore, Chase and Mandle 2001). I collected data from multiple groups (e.g., families, people with dementia, clinicians, Non-Government Organization [NGO] workers and government officials) and have compared and contrasted their views throughout this book. I observed in clinical settings and families' homes as well as in the broader community. Representations of caregiving in government documents, medical bodies and film narratives have been analysed (see Brijnath and Manderson 2008). These methods, when compiled, provide a complex montage that expiates the differences between how care *should* be given and how it *is* given.

My Spiritual Museum for Character Building

Data were collected in Delhi, augmented with brief work undertaken in Kolkata, Bangalore and parts of Kerala. I also travelled to smaller north Indian cities like Dehradun, Amritsar and Jaipur. During these trips I interviewed key service providers, observed caregiving in different contexts and gained insight into the multiplicity of Indian societies by geography. Sometimes my journeys to these cities began just as an escape from Delhi.

In total I spent 9.5 months in Delhi and 10.10 months in India. I selected Delhi as the principal field site for a number of reasons: the cultural pluralities of the city, my familiarity with the surroundings and the paucity of research work on ageing in this region since the late 1990s (see Vatuk 1990; Van Willigen and Chadha 1999). Much of the work on dementia in India has been undertaken by members or affiliates of the 10/66 Dementia Research Group, an international network of over 100 researchers (Prince et al. 2004). In India, their work has been concentrated in the western and southern regions, in places such as Goa, Kerala and Tamil Nadu. Many 10/66 researchers reside in these states and have established links with the Alzheimer's and Related Disorders Society of India (ARDSI), which supports people with dementia (discussed later). During the course of my fieldwork, ARDSI Chapters in the south and west were better resourced than their northern counterparts and it was easier to mobilize participants and conduct research on dementia in these areas. By way of example, nine of the twelve epidemiological studies undertaken to ascertain the prevalence of dementia have been undertaken in these regions. The north and east of India are relatively unexplored.

Delhi and north India differ markedly from the rest of the country because of variations in language, local economies, education, politics and the role of women. With a population of 16.7 million people, Delhi is the largest urban agglomeration in India (Census of India 2011). The city is part of the National Capital Region (NCR), approximately 33,000sq. km of conurbation that includes parcels of land from neighbouring states Uttar Pradesh, Haryana and Rajasthan (National Capital Region Planning Board 2010). Currently 7.6 per cent of India's urban population resides in the NCR alone and population density in the region has more than doubled in the last three decades from 657 persons per sq.km in 1981 to 1349 persons per sq.km in 2011 (the national average was 382 persons per sq.km in 2011) (National Capital Region Planning Board 2010).

The genesis of the NCR can be traced to the Delhi Master Plan of 1962, where, in order to alleviate pressures on existing resources, nearby villages were rapidly industrialized to become satellite cities (Overview of the National Capital Region 2010). However, the agglomeration trend has even older roots. Since the fifteenth century, Delhi has been the site of empires built, conquered, abandoned, plundered and rebuilt. The city is said to comprise seven cities – Quila Rai Pithora, Mehrauli, Siri, Tughlakabad, Firozabad, Shergarh and Shahjehabanad – and is often dubbed a 'city of cities' (Vidal, Tarlo and Dupont 2000).

More recent additions to Delhi's metropolis include Gurgaon, Noida, Faridabad and Ghaziabad. In close proximity to Delhi, these locales are linked via public transport, commuters flow across the borders on a daily basis and there is little difference between them and 'old' Delhi in terms of urbanization. There are of course differences according to socio-economic status.[1]

Delhi's growth can be attributed to the influx of people from other parts of India, especially the neighbouring states of Haryana, Punjab, Rajasthan and Uttar Pradesh. Young people, mostly men, come to Delhi in search of employment in the formal and informal labour economies, while women migrate predominantly for marriage and as part of migrating families (Dupont 2000). In 2004, young people under twenty-five years constituted the majority of the population (49.48 per cent) but the proportion of people over the age of sixty years has also been shown to be increasing;[2] approximately 829,000 people in Delhi are over the age of sixty, about 5.5 per cent of the population (in 2001 the percentage was 5.2) (Government of National Capital Territory of Delhi 2006). Older people aged sixty to sixty-nine years comprise 65.68 per cent of the older people in Delhi, thus making the population relatively young-old (Government of National Capital Territory of Delhi 2006). Just over half (51.8 per cent) live with their spouse and children, a third (27.6 per cent) without their children,

14.4 per cent without their spouse and only with their children and the remainder live with others (whether extended family or friends). Of those who live alone or with their spouse, nearly 40 per cent live in the same building as their children, 28.5 per cent live in the same area and about 30 per cent live in another town or village (Government of National Capital Territory of Delhi 2006). In total around 66 per cent of older Delhi-ites live with their children and of the remainder that do not, nearly 70 per cent either reside in the same building or nearby.[3] Such figures reflect standard household living arrangements across India and indicate that cohabitation between older parents and an adult child and/or adult children supporting older parents is common in India.

Moreover, 70 per cent of the aged in Delhi are financially supported by their children, 22 per cent rely on their spouse, a marginal 2.7 per cent look to their grandchildren for financial aid and 4 per cent are supported by others (Government of National Capital Territory of Delhi 2006). Thus despite the 'perils' of modernity, it appears that families have adapted and found ways to support and live within pseudo joint family systems in urban environments.

Although it is the fastest growing city in India, Delhi is renowned for inspiring indifference and dislike on the part of many of its residents (Vidal et al. 2000). Even the city's longest serving Chief Minister, Sheila Dixit, described Delhi as 'The most crass and show-offish city of the current times' (Dixit cited in Soofi 2008). Personal safety is a key issue, contributing to the city's reputation as hard and dangerous. Such perceptions are borne out by statistics: in 2008, when I collected my data, 22.4 per cent of all reported rape cases, 30.5 per cent of kidnappings, 15.3 per cent of dowry deaths and 15.4 per cent of all reported molestation cases in Indian cities occurred in Delhi (NCRB 2008).

Growing up in Kolkata (1982–1993) and Delhi (1993–2000), I recall Delhi as an aggressive city publicly overlaid by a kind of hypermasculinity and consumerism. As a teenager and then as a young woman, I remember having to manage not only my own body and sexuality, but also those of the men around me when I went out. 'Eve-teasing' (verbal and physical harassment) on the street was commonplace. When I returned in 2008, I anticipated similar experiences. My worst fears were realized when I began to look for a place to stay. Many housing agents showed me horrible places and landlords were quick to establish extra terms and conditions upon discovering that I would be living alone. Some wanted me to be 'pure vegetarian', others to impose a curfew and have me home by 10:30P.M. or else remain locked out all night; still others would permit neither houseguests nor visitors, with the exception of my parents or close female friends.

These tactics were irritating and a huge blow to my feminist heart. They seemed to confirm my worst assumptions about how women were perceived. But as time went by, I realized that the city had changed in the near decade since I had moved away. We had both matured, becoming stronger and less aggressive. The eve-teasers had dropped off in numbers and life seemed a little less Hobbesian than before. As I gallivanted around this uneasy city by myself, earning the nickname *Ghumantru* (wanderer) from ARDSI staff, I felt safer than I ever had in the past. Post-fieldwork, as the sweet glaze of nostalgia overlays my memories, I see the city as part of my character building.

I also soon came to realize that the extra terms that landlords laid on me reflected local ideas of morality, femininity and tenancy and are embedded in a discourse of reciprocity and kinship. The standard line often went: '*Beta* (child), you will be like a daughter in this house. Anybody can come and go, no problem – but no boys'. While these terms were neither equal nor fair, in these reciprocal relations, I did come to be daughter in many houses and *didi* (older sister) in others. Claiming kinship is common in India. People are connected to each other through terms of address like *bhaiya:* (brother), *didi* and *mātāji* (mother). Being connected is important because through such networks all manner of activities, legal and illicit, transpire. Class, gender, age, social capital, income, ethnicity and education are implicit within this paradigm. In Delhi, one must be connected, whether by fair means or foul and in a city of millions, though one may sometimes be lonely, one is never alone.

I eventually found a place to live in a steamy *barsathi* (two rooms on a terrace) in south Delhi. My landlord, Mr Papneja senior, who I called 'sir', though initially uninterested in forging kinship alliances, inevitably became family. I often found myself babysitting his great grandchildren during their summer holidays and being fed *ghee-parathas* by his wife, whom I called *mātāji*. When I was not around, my mail and my ironing would be left in their house; and when I ran terrified from the lizards, Papneja senior installed a mesh screen on my windows. I came to know the family quite well – Sir and his wife *Mātāji*, their son and daughter-in-law Kuku and Sheelu, their grandchildren Summi, Aditya and Vicky and their great grandchildren, Neeti, Suresh and Noddy.

The *barsathi* was my haven, tucked in the bottom of the lane with only a silk-cotton tree for company (see Fig. 1.1). However, as the heat increased, more residents arrived – lizards, ants, bees, birds, mosquitoes, an assortment of other bugs and the occasional cat. By summer, the vegetable prices had soared, cold water came out of the hot water tap because the water in the geyser was cooler than the water in the tank and the fans whirled relentlessly. The *loo* began to sweep through the city and these dust storms

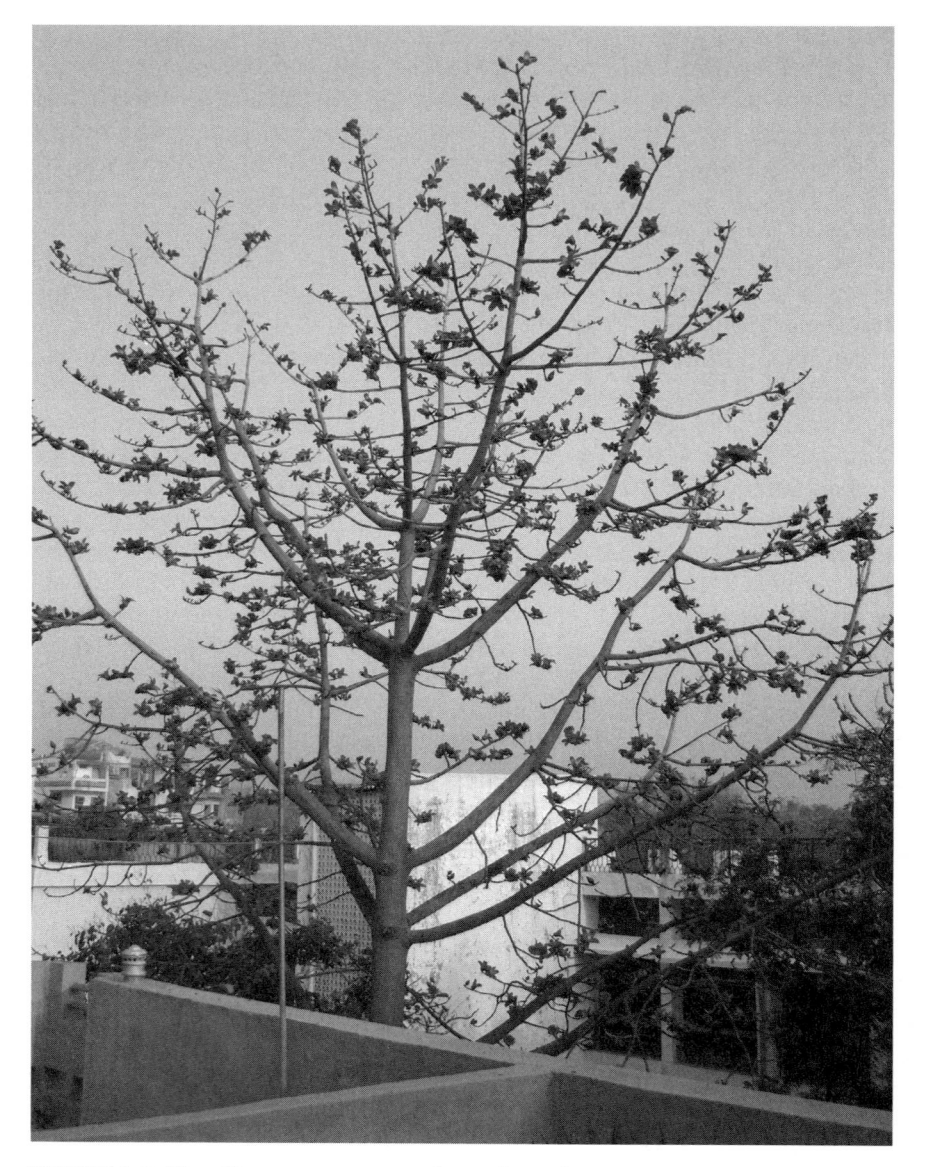

FIGURE 1.1 The silk-cotton tree outside my *barsathi*

exacerbated the existing dust, turning clear 43-degree skies grey-blue and the vegetation brown.

Only the inner sanctums of the city, enclosed between the Inner Ring Road and Connaught Place in south Delhi, remained gorgeous. Diplomats, politicians, senior government officials and 'old money' lived there on wide, spotless roads, behind guarded green fences. For these people, seasonal changes brought with them few alterations in lifestyle – they were buffered against power cuts, water shortages and the blistering heat by their political and literal connections to generators, water tanks and air conditioners. These Delhi elite easily switched from pegs of whisky and polo-necks in winter to gin and linen *kurta:s* in summer. The rest struggled with chronic electricity and water shortages and were grubby in their vests and shorts.

Amidst the inequality and heat, the city does have some redeeming features, also noted by others (see Dalrymple 1994; Singh 1989). As Delhi is the political capital of India, ministries, public offices, headquarters of national airlines, railways, census boards and archives are located here. Media empires are clustered here alongside major universities, corporations and hospitals, including the widely regarded All India Institute of Medical Sciences (Cadène 2000). I visited many of these sites as I collected data. There were also film festivals, playhouses and old friends to keep me company. The construction of metropolitan railways, shopping centres, highways and bus lanes gave the city movement, helped along by the unceasing traffic (see Fig. 1.2). The din floated into my *barsathi* every evening, along with the tunes of the latest Bollywood hit, *Mauja*,

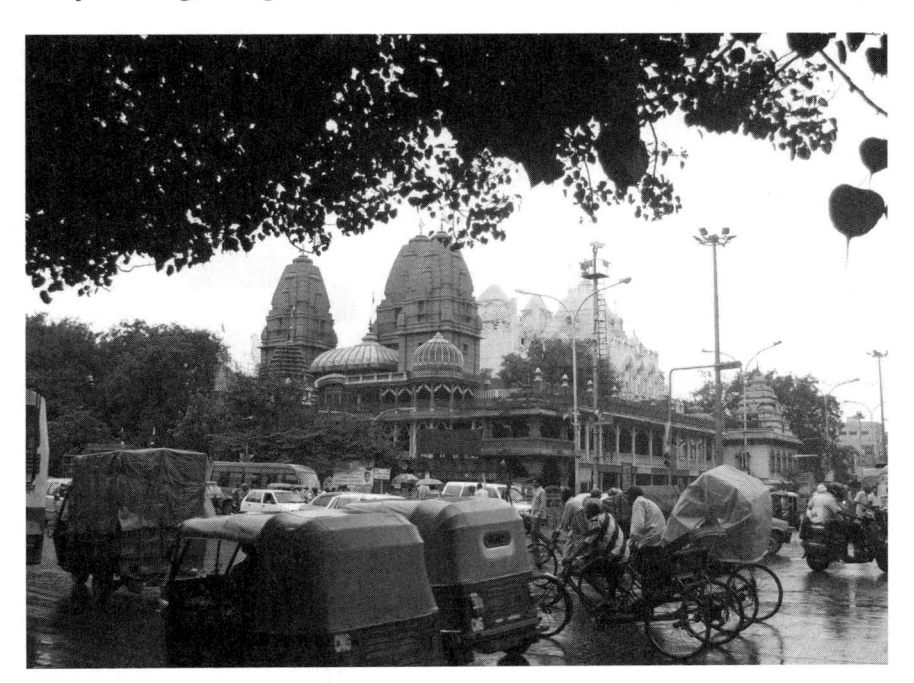

FIGURE 1.2 Delhi on the move

Mauja! (naughty fun). During this time the lizards and I battled it out for supremacy over the terrace. I repeatedly lost.

The Alzheimer's and Related Disorders Society of India (ARDSI)

I recruited my participants through the Alzheimer's and Related Disorders Society of India, Delhi Chapter (ARDSI-DC). The advantages of working with ARDSI were fourfold: (1) people with dementia were already clinically screened and diagnosed; (2) families had a pre-existing relationship with biomedicine and were able to comment on the quality of treatment; (3) ARDSI's volunteers worked closely with people with dementia and their carers and had knowledge of the family's history, which assisted in identifying potential participants; and (4) ARDSI was there to provide support to families should they become distressed during the research and was able to act as a source for any complaints about the research process (though fortunately neither happened). This approach strengthened the collaborative process and introduced a measure of transparency and accountability to participants.

ARDSI was established in 1992 by Dr Jacob Roy and a number of other doctors, most of who come from Kerala in south India. At the time of writing (2013), Dr Roy is still chairman, the head office recently moved from Kochi, Kerala to Delhi and the ARDSI Board still comprises many original members, mostly neurologists and psychiatrists. The aims of the organization are to provide information and services for people with dementia and their families across India. These aims are in line with the goals of Alzheimer's Disease International, an umbrella organization of national Alzheimer's associations throughout the world, of which ARDSI is a member. ARDSI has sixteen Chapters based in cities across India and offers a range of services such as day care, domiciliary care, geriatric care training, caregivers' meetings and guidance and counselling. However, not all services are available at every Chapter, because each Chapter has to provide its own funds and is reliant on local donations and the goodwill of volunteers. Paid staff and continuity of funds are scarce and this impacts on each Chapter's capacity to offer services (ARDSI 2006).

In approaching ARDSI, I first sought the support of the chairman Dr Roy, when I met him at the 2007 Alzheimer's Australia Annual Conference in Perth. In this early conversation, we tried to map how ARDSI could help, but because I was dealing with the semi-autonomous Delhi Chapter, this was never entirely clear. Once I arrived in Delhi, the incumbent ARDSI Delhi president gave me a list of tasks with the gentle caveat, 'Perform or be on the periphery and redundant'. Fortunately this ultimatum was in line with the services I had planned to volunteer and so these demands were not onerous. I found myself writing newsletters, filling log books, mobilizing volunteers, assisting with functions, preparing grant submissions and dispensing strategic advice. I gained insight into how the organization functioned – the office politics, finances and quality of service delivery.

The Delhi Chapter was small, staffed only by three workers paid via donation, a handful of dedicated volunteers and a quixotic president. It was sustained through material and monetary donations. In 2008, two old computers, floppy disks and one cranky printer were the only technical equipment available. The volunteers were in their fifties and sixties and came from affluent backgrounds. The women tended to be housewives and the men semi-retired. Often their children and grandchildren were married and settled elsewhere. Working for an NGO was one amongst many activities pursued, like kitty parties,[4] book clubs and golf. There were a few disgruntled key service providers who perceived these volunteers as 'high society ladies' dabbling in charitable endeavours. But based on my own observation there could be little doubt of their hard work and commitment. Volunteers travelled long distances across Delhi in heat, traffic and dust; they bullied, cajoled and wheedled funds from their rich friends to donate to ARDSI; and they gave generously of their own money and possessions (air conditioners, computers, tables, chairs, curtains, examining tables and so on). Many had parents or friends who had died from Alzheimer's disease. Some had been carers and recipients of ARDSI services prior to joining as volunteers and these people were especially dedicated.

At ARDSI-DC, free medicines were dispensed to poor people, the volunteers trained women living in slums to become home care attendants (see Fig. 1.3) and awareness-raising sessions took place in low-income neighbourhoods. But by and large, the membership consisted of middle-class families and common social understandings of class between the volunteers and families enabled volunteers to most effectively counsel these families. These families were also most likely to attend caregivers' meetings and champion their rights. Poorer families had neither the inclination nor the resources to travel to ARDSI-DC's office. They would not attend functions such as World Alzheimer's Day or ARDSI-DC's Founders Day. For them, the locations of these events, in elite parts of south Delhi, were barriers themselves. The need for ARDSI-DC to expand its purview to better include poorer families was recognized by people within the NGO. The Delhi Chapter President and staff began to forge partnerships with other organizations that worked with lower-income groups. When I left, these relationships were in their infancy but I have little doubt that with more money, mature partnerships and professionalization, the organization will achieve great things.

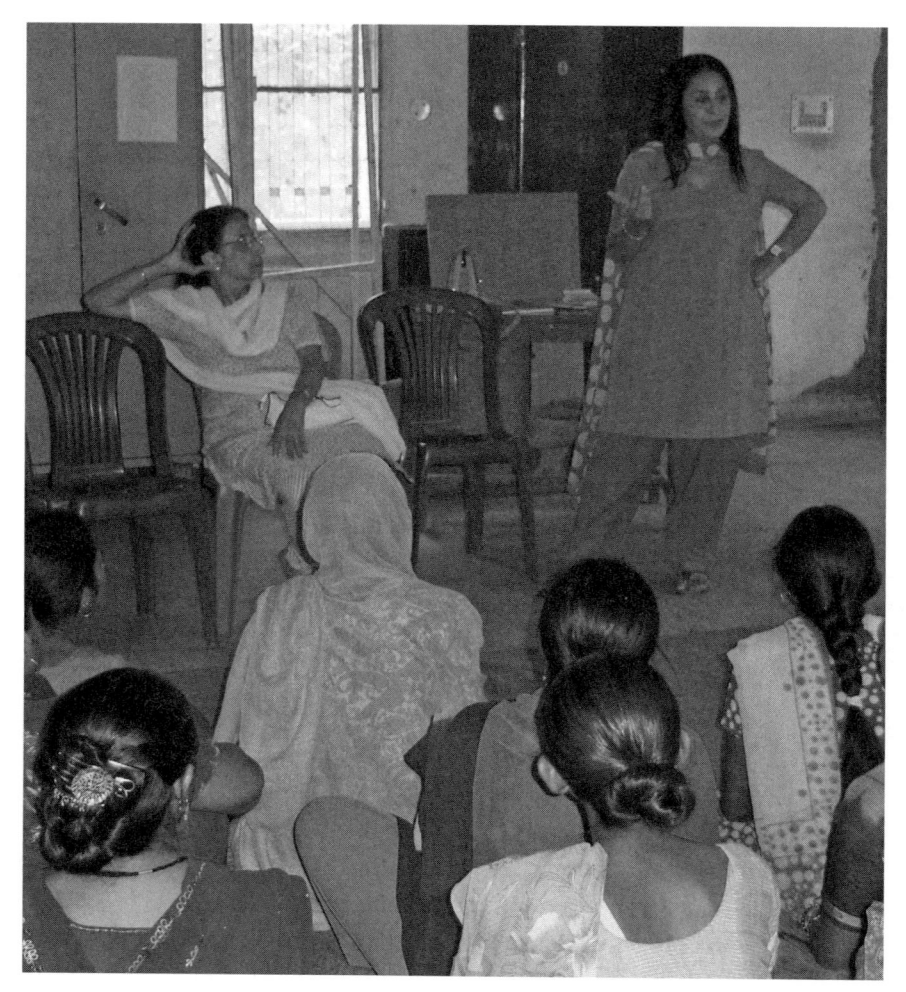

FIGURE 1.3 ARDSI volunteers training poor women to be home attendants

Participants

The Families

Families caring for people with dementia were members of ARDSI-DC who had been recruited via volunteers. I accompanied volunteers on visits to people's homes (n=13 families recruited), attended official functions and meetings (n=4 families recruited) and spent many hours in two public hospital Out Patient Departments (OPDs) (n=3 families recruited). These OPD sessions also functioned as ARDSI-DC 'Memory Clinics' on designated days. The two doctors, who ran the OPDs in their respective hospitals, were well known specialists and board members of ARDSI-DC. They gave me permission to observe in their consultation rooms and from their referrals, I managed to recruit three families.

Face-to-face contact was critical to successful recruitment. In six cases, volunteers had obtained consent over the telephone from families to pass their details onto me. Despite repeated follow up and explanation about my project, these interviews never occurred. People would indirectly rescind through claims of not having enough time, household renovations and preoccupation with other tasks. If I was put off twice, I would remind people of my mobile number and ask them to contact me when they were available. None ever did. Conversely, those with whom I had face-to-face contact gave consent and made time for our interview soon after. These early meetings were an important opportunity for potential participants to judge me, establish a rapport and ask questions about the project and my personal life.

In total, forty-six interviews were conducted with twenty families over ten months. The sample was relatively cross-sectional: there were seventeen Hindu families and one family each who were Christian, Muslim and Sikh. Thirteen families were from north India (e.g., Punjab, Uttar Pradesh, Kashmir), four from south India (e.g., Kerala, Andhra Pradesh), one from West Bengal and two Punjabi families had migrated from Pakistan during Partition.[5] Geographically the families were spread across Delhi; eight families lived in south Delhi (including Gurgaon), seven in the west (including Dwarka), four in the east (including Ghaziabad and Noida) and one in the north.

Given the composition of the ARDSI-DC database, the majority of families were middle class (n=15), the remainder affluent (n=5). Ascertaining monthly income was not viable because many carers had retired and relied on their children and/or pensions for financial support and so their monthly incomes fluctuated considerably. In my observations, wealthy families tended to live in bungalows or large apartments in very exclusive suburbs. They had chauffeurs who drove their Japanese or German cars, holidayed annually or biannually in places like Europe or Singapore and had additional rental properties elsewhere in the city along with share and investment portfolios. Middle-class families lived in apartments in colonies, usually had one modest hatchback that they drove themselves, holidayed within India or nearby Bangkok and tended not to discuss their additional assets (if they had any). Among those who were in the middle-class bracket, three families were lower middle class and struggled to make ends meet; the rest were financially stable. Those who struggled were thrifty – they rarely went to the movies or shopped for new clothes, they took buses rather than auto-rickshaws and they often bought diapers and medicines on credit. For example, Suneeta Sadhwani (41) would bring her seventy-four-year-old father with dementia to the ARDSI-DC office on a crowded bus, because she could not afford the Rs 70 (A$1.70) it would cost to come via auto-rickshaw.

Caste was not cited by any of the families and in my observations, the vertical interdependence of caste did not appear to explicitly structure families' interactions with the wider community. Dumont's (1980) *Homo Hierarchicus*, with its strict accounts of purity and pollution, seemed well and truly displaced by other measures of inequity such as wealth, income, education and occupation. Such findings have been reiterated in other studies, which also note the increased competition among caste groups for limited political and economic resources (see Ali 2002; Beteille 1997; Fuller 1996).

Among those I interviewed, there were more men with dementia than women (n=12 to n=8; mean age 76.05 years). Epidemiological findings from urban India reveal that dementia is associated with increases in age but not gender (Shaji, Bose and Verghese 2005; Vas et al. 2001). In line with the feminization of care, the primary carers were mostly women (n=17; mean age 52.65 years), including the wives (n=7), daughters (n=6) and daughters-in-law (n=4) of the person with dementia. This does not mean that men played no role in caregiving, rather that they assumed more supportive or secondary roles. But even here, women almost doubled men as secondary carers (n=11 women to n=5 men).

Categorizing family members into primary and secondary carers is problematic, however, because in some families, more than one person saw himself or herself as primary caregiver. In the Sen-Hamdari-Kaul family, for example, Kumud Kaul lived above her parents, Mr and Mrs Hamdari, and would oversee the cooking, cleaning and the care of her mother, Mrs Hamdari (who had dementia). Nayantara Sen, Kumud's younger sister, lived a short distance away but visited her parents every day to supervise the administration of medications, check the medical supplies, organize refills and accompany her mother to doctor's appointments. Mr Hamdari, though responsible for almost no aspects of his wife's care, spent all day with her and knew the most about her personality and mood swings. To categorize their efforts as primary, secondary or even tertiary would diminish the important work each person performed and undermine the collective nature of the care given to Mrs Hamdari. Nevertheless I have arbitrarily coded one family member into each category to compile basic demographic information about the overall sample. This has been done for easy understanding of the relations between families and has only been mapped so deterministically in Table 1. In the remainder of the book, such

TABLE 1.1 Demographic data of families (pseudonyms have been used)

No.	PED* Name	PED age	PED's PC^	PC name	PC age	PED's SC§	SC name	SC age
1.	Mrs Meenakshi Ranjarajan	78	Daughter	Mrs Parvati Gowda	43	Son	Mr Gopal Ranjarajan	–
2.	Mr Rajesh Kumar Menon	71	Wife	Mrs Radha Menon	61	Daughter	Mrs Rajni	–
3.	Mr Sudhanshu Talwar	78	Daughter-in-law	Mrs Savitri Talwar	–	Son	Mr Hemant Talwar	
4.	Mrs Helen Meena Chand	82	Husband	Mr Shivbaksh Chand	85	–		–
5.	Mrs Meera Chopra	80	Husband	Mr Kundan Lal (K.L.) Chopra	88	Daughter-in-law	Mrs Rubina Chopra	–
6.	Mr K.P. Aggarwal	69	Wife	Mrs Sita Aggarwal	63	Daughter-in-law	Mrs Mamta Aggarwal	–
7.	Mrs Lakshmi Kumari Kochar	92	Daughter-in-law	Mrs Sarojini Kochar	69	Attendant	Ms Sonu	21
8.	Mr C.K. Sethi	81	Daughter-in-law	Mrs Chandana Sethi	–	Wife	Mrs Sonali Sethi	–
9.	Mr S.T. Pillai	87	Daughter	Ms Nandini Pillai	52	–		–
10.	Mrs Tara Jaiswal	85	Daughter	Mrs Bhageshwari Srivastava	41	Daughter	Ms Gayatri	–
11.	Mr Gautam Mukherjee	88	Wife	Mrs Shilpi Mukherjee	72	Attendant	Mrs Sandra Anu	39
12.	Mr A.P. Arora	79	Daughter-in-law	Mrs Vandhana Arora	38	Wife	Mrs Mrigakshi Arora	74
13.	Mr Hari Prasad Sadhwani	74	Daughter	Ms Suneeta Sadhwani	41	–		–
14.	Mrs Sheila Tandon	58	Husband	Mr Govind Ballabh Tandon	58	Attendant	Ms Payal	22
15.	Mr Karamjit Bhagat	75	Wife	Mrs Nina Bhagat	70	Son	Mr Vikram Bhagat	–
16.	Mrs Shanti Hamdari	80	Daughter	Mrs Nayantara Sen	58	Daughter	Mrs Kumud Kaul	60
17.	Mr Surinder Dharam Singh	56	Wife	Mrs Josephine (Josie) Dharam Singh	52	Attendant	Mr Santosh	–
18.	Mr Harinder Singh	60	Wife	Mrs Jaspreet Kaur	55	Son	Mr Ajit Singh	28
19.	Mr Omar Khan	65	Wife	Mrs Shafia Khan	54	Son	Mr Naseer Khan	21
20.	Mrs Anjeli Sood	83	Daughter	Ms Namita Sood	53	Daughter	Ms Aditi Sood	–

Notes: * PED = Person experiencing dementia   ^ PC = Primary carer   § SC = Secondary carer distinctions have not been made. All names and identifying details have been changed to protect participants' anonymity.

Key Service Providers (KSPs)

I have defined a key service provider as any person providing in a formal capacity direct health, care or social support to people with dementia and their families. Initial participants were recruited via purposive sampling and from there, snowballing techniques were used. Interviews (n=21) were conducted in Delhi, Kolkata, Kochi and Bangalore with clinicians, NGO workers, paid attendants, government officials and the police. Most KSPs had dual responsibilities such as working in a medical practice and for an NGO or government department. For example, ten KSPs had a clinical qualification and six of these were also members of ARDSI. Additionally, there were more male KSPs than women (twelve and nine respectively) and men tended to have much higher positions of authority than women (e.g., of ten clinicians, seven were men and three women).

Procedures

Interviews were semi-structured and while broadly focused on dementia care, questions were adjusted according to participants' background and settings. For example, police were not asked about diagnosis, management and prognosis of dementia, just as clinicians were not queried about crimes against older people. All KSPs were asked about the impact of gender, caste, class and income on families' health-seeking behaviours, the role of stigma (if applicable) in lay perceptions of dementia, the support systems available and the barriers (if any) that families and KSPs encountered when accessing such systems. Interviews with KSPs and family members were generally about one hour long, after informed consent had been received. Where permission was granted, interviews were recorded and transcribed. KSP interviews were conducted in their workplaces and all interviews with families took place in their homes.

Non-participant observation was undertaken in some KSPs' workplaces, i.e. two government hospital Out Patient Departments (OPDs) in Delhi. With the permission of hospital clinicians, I attended these OPDs to observe standard clinical care practices for people with dementia, doctor-patient communication and the effect various factors – such as time, patient load, multiple work demands and the availability of resources – had on these processes. Each observation session was approximately two hours and detailed field notes were taken immediately after I left. Approximately twenty-one hours of observation were undertaken, spread over ten months.

Topics covered with families included diagnosis, treatment, management of symptoms, pleasures and difficulties of carework, experiences with neighbours, friends and broader society and changing relationships within the home. While interviews with families tended to last for approximately an hour, each visit to their home lasted between two to four hours. During this time participant observation was undertaken, meals were shared and friendships built. I noted how carers and people with dementia experienced care in the private familial setting, the routines, restrictions and negotiations around particular activities, communication strategies and techniques of containment. I had initially planned to follow the non-participant observation approach used by Briggs and colleagues (2007, 2003) in their work on dementia care, at home, in England. But I quickly realized (as they did) that becoming 'part of the furniture' during observation in such settings is impossible. While Briggs' participants tolerated and sometimes even forgot the researcher's presence, my arrival in people's homes was an occasion, marked by food, conversation and in the early days, a carnivalesque atmosphere. The first time I went to interview Chandhana Sethi, her two sisters-in-law, mother-in-law and father-in-law were there during the interview. Tea, biscuits and sweets were served, everyone wanted to be recorded and MRIs and medical histories were pulled from dusty cupboards. Similarly, in my second interview with Shivbaksh Chand, a friend from the local health dispensary across the street was called to witness and participate in our interview.

Once I became aware of the carnival, and therefore the gravitas, of my interviews with families, I knew non-participant methods would not work. A more organic stance had to be embraced, which offered space for multiple realities, playfulness, irony, pastiche and parody (Grbich 2007). I often found that my interviews and observations did not go to plan, neither did they conform to any textbook prescriptions on how to do an interview. What I thought would happen rarely did. Instead there were three distinctive features that disrupted traditional interview paradigms: (1) people's assumption that I was a medical doctor; (2) the lack of privacy and frequent interruptions during the interview; and (3) the unique ways in which consent was given for the participation of people with dementia in this study. I will deal with each of these in turn.

'Madam Has Come, the Doctor Has Come'

By doing research on a health related subject, I was often assumed to be either a medical doctor or, at least, a medical student. Accordingly an array of health problems and information were presented to me: leg pain, back pain, weakness, depression, heart problems, MRIs, X-rays and test results. Despite my telling people that I was not a doctor, they persisted in treating me as such.

Such behaviour cut across gender, age and education. Lower middle-class people would typically call me 'doctor *sāhib*' (doctor sir) or 'madam', as they told me in graphic, unsolicited detail about their various ailments. Higher-income groups would address me by name rather than as 'doctor', but implicitly assumed that I had a wealth of medical knowledge that could help to alleviate all kinds of distress. Specifically with respect to dementia, families would frequently ask how they should understand the dementia diagnosis, manage medication, deal with difficult behaviours (such as violence, incontinence, paranoia and sleeplessness), what to do in palliative care and how to treat comorbidities (like cataract, diabetes and diarrhoea).

Initially such questions caused me considerable anxiety and numerous referrals were made to doctors and NGO workers. To me, these questions signalled a lack of awareness about dementia and reflected the poor communication between doctors, NGOs and people. Yet I persisted in referring people to health services, convinced this was the only ethical way to proceed. After a while, such referrals came to seem foolish. If health services had consistently failed to communicate effectively, then sending people back there again and again, with neither new information nor confidence to ask new questions, was a waste of their time and health services resources. I had to be more proactive in assisting families and to intervene directly in some cases. The Indian health system is hierarchical and a 'researcher' has more access, acceptability and authority with a doctor than patients or their families. So I began to accompany many families to the doctor, made suggestions to them at home and functioned as a source for them to express their frustrations. I never dispensed medical advice but in some cases – such as where drug dosages for antipsychotics had remained unchanged for over three years – I would encourage carers to go to their doctor and ask purposely about these practices.

I also came to realize that people addressed me as 'doctor *sāhib*' not just because they conflated medicine and medical anthropology, but also because it was a way to show respect. People generally had deep admiration for doctors and those who were called 'doctor *sāhib*' were located in a biomedical paradigm. In traditional medical frameworks, practitioners are more likely to be referred to as '*vaidji*' or '*ḥakīmji*'. In calling me 'doctor *sāhib*', families situated me in the biomedical camp. This was further cemented by my transnational background (Indian-Australian), high levels of education and ease with the English language. Families were appreciative of the efforts I made to understand their perspectives, some perhaps a little too much, such as the Chopra family, who tried to pay me Rs 500 for interviewing them! They were only dissuaded after I promised teary-eyed Kundan Lal that I would return and accept *prasād* (food that is blessed) from their local temple.

The Interrupted Interview

In this study there was no such thing as an uninterrupted interview. Phone calls, visitors, cooking and household chores always occurred simultaneously. In doctor's clinics, patients, files and consultations were all dealt with at the same time as the interview. Interviews were frequently paused and an hour of tape could sometimes take two hours to record. In one case, a KSP halted our interview midway to dash off to a conference and we were only able to resume our conversation the following week.

In addition, there were a number of surprise additions to the interviews. Participants would brief their colleagues, friends or extended family about the research project and invite them to participate. I was never informed about these additional subjects, who would often arrive halfway through the interview, sometimes to participate and at other times to observe. Occasionally the person with whom I had arranged the interview would get up and leave halfway and this secondary person would enter as the new subject and keep the conversation going.

Trying to obtain prior informed consent from these secondary voices under such circumstances was not possible. Rather than disrupt the interview to brief them on the project and get their consent, I would silently check with them that I could use the tape recorder. Once the entire interview had concluded, then I would brief these participants on the project and ask if they were happy to participate or have their contributions excluded from the transcript. None rescinded.

But while people were happy to give verbal consent, publicly disclose medical histories (whether solicited or not) and reveal body parts, there was a profound distrust of written consent. Irrespective of their education and life experiences, people did not want to sign the consent form. None of the families and few KSPs agreed to sign. The documents were perceived as threatening, with potential legal ramifications. In one of my interviews with a clinician (who also has a research profile), a legal representative, dubbed a 'well-wisher', was present during the interview. The representative only left once the participant was assured that he did not have to sign the consent form. Participants' unwillingness to sign consent forms also highlights different notions of consent and researcher-participant relations as compared to Western countries. Researchers have noted that consent in many developing nations tends to be collective, follows from extensive consultation and is perceived as an opportunity to build relations between researchers and participants over time (Gikonyo et al. 2008; Marshall 2006). Communities in the Asia-Pacific region hold to these ideas and colleagues and I have described the dissonance between ethical review processes in Australia and the challenges of obtaining consent in this part of the world (see Czymoniewicz-Klippel, Brijnath and Crockett 2010).

The Failed Protocol

There is increased criticism of ethics committees and research projects that focus on dementia but exclude the participation of people living with this disease (see Bartlett and Martin 2002; Dewing 2007; Hellstrom et al. 2007; Swain, Heyman and Gillman 1998). However, in my initial research design, I did not intend to actively recruit people with dementia. Trying to shape a path that gave voice to the experiences of people living with dementia, while building in safety nets in the event that they became distressed, was not straightforward. In India, there is a documented lack of proper medical care and little formal support; the onus rests entirely on the family. The challenge was how to include caregivers and people living with dementia into the project, while satisfying the university's Ethics Committee's requirements to minimize participant distress and do no harm in what were inherently distressing situations.

Thus a complicated procedure was developed: first the person with dementia had to initiate contact with their primary carer and/or me to express their desire to be interviewed. Then the primary carer had to agree and abide by a 'Protocol to Minimize Interview Distress for People with Dementia'. The protocol involved the following: after the primary caregiver gave permission to access the person with dementia, the basis for consent was to be established by identifying the usual presentation of the person with dementia and, more importantly, the early signs of distress. The time and place where initial consent was given was to be recorded. Then, the interview would commence with ongoing monitoring for signs of distress or withdrawal of consent. The primary caregiver (who in theory could see but not hear the interview) was also to be engaged in this monitoring and, finally, debriefing and provision of feedback and support for both the person with dementia and the caregiver was to be offered by me (if necessary). The protocol echoed Dewing's (2007) 'Process Consent Method',[6] but lacked the organic seamlessness of her approach and relied too much on the participation of the carer and not the person with dementia. If the former declined to assist, then the interview with the latter could not proceed. The protocol actually risked excluding people with dementia.

In practice the Protocol was ineffective and never used. There are two reasons for this: (1) issues in identifying the primary caregiver; and (2) caregivers' use of my presence to validate themselves as 'good' caregivers and 'good' human beings. I have already discussed how categorizing people as primary and secondary caregivers was problematic because multiple people saw themselves in these roles. Such sharing of responsibilities, though common, made it difficult to identify from whom to seek permission to access the person living with dementia.

More importantly people with dementia were immediately accessible to me when I visited families' homes. There was no opportunity for them to approach me and express a desire to be interviewed; instead people with dementia were bathed, powdered, perfumed and dressed in their good clothes before I had arrived. Those who were mobile would often be seated in their living rooms or would otherwise be propped up in bed. Families would insist I meet and talk to the person with dementia immediately. Then they would demand a response from me on the appearance and character of their loved one. I was frequently asked, 'How does he or she seem to you?' These practices were part of the heuristic techniques used to manage images of normality, disruption and mitigate stigma (see Chapter 6).

Initially these displays were confronting and in the early days I would stammer to find a neutral answer. Later, as my relationships grew stronger with families, I was more forthright. I realized if I was to be 'doctor *sāhib*', then I might as well use this power and authority to effect some change, rather than simply collecting stories of care and only offering recommendations in a book many years later. So in these later interactions, I gave advice about additional medical consultations, new activities to pass the time together and offers to accompany people to the clinic.

Consent from caregivers to talk with the person with dementia was often rooted in a need for self-validation rather than research altruism. Caring could be lonely and exhausting, with neither adequate feedback from healthcare professionals nor wider social support. And while caregivers, by putting their patients on display and inviting me to engage with the person with dementia, gave consent to these interactions, people with dementia either consented or rescinded in their own fashion. They would, either verbally or through their body language, indicate disinterest and an unwillingness to participate. I will expand on some of these tactics in Chapter 7 when I describe how I learnt to listen to what people with dementia were telling me.

Professional and Personal Ethics

Ethical ways of doing research can be classified roughly into two categories – institutional (formal) and personal (informal) (Guillemin and Gillam 2004). In a formal sense, I obtained approval for the study from Monash University Human Research Ethics Committee, the Alzheimer's and Related Disorders Society of India and the Government of India, which, upon issuing me with my Overseas Citizen of India visa, advised that no further research clearance would be required.

In the field, my ethics were constantly tested. In what I did (or did not do), I was not always who I like to think I am. The personal and the professional did not match; neither did the rhetoric and practice. Instead I found myself in what McLean and Leibing (2007) so evocatively call 'the shadow side of fieldwork', that ambiguous topography, full of light and shadow that frames how we view the field and our practices within it.

But if the intent is 'seeing what frames our seeing' (Davies et al. 2004: 364), then I need to further elucidate my position in this research. In the field, I never shied away from discussing my grandmother and our family's experiences, but I did not seek to base my relations with my participants on such foundations. In subsequent analysis, I have tried very hard not to overlay my own caregiving experiences on those of my participants. While there can be little doubt that my experience and that of my family of caring for our grandmother shaped my analysis and affected my relations with participants, this book is very explicitly about the experiences of these families who I came to know in Delhi and not about my personal experience of caregiving.

Lastly, I worked hard to build empathy and trust with all my participants, yet I cannot say that I became friends with them. My youth, gender and worldview in an urban, conservative, north Indian environment proved strong barriers (even though I tried hard to shut up and blend in most of the time). But I did build intimacy. The depth of connection between families and myself, forged at its own natural pace, emerging organically and in the intimacies of friendship (not researcher-subject), echoes what Tillmann-Healy (2003) describes as 'friendship as method'. These have made the stories rich and I am privileged to have shared them.

Analysis – Can You Smell the Writing?

Interviews were conducted in Hindi and English, tape recorded, then translated and transcribed in English and imported into NVivo ver.8 for coding and thematic analyses. A similar process of transcription and data management was followed for the field notes. All identifying features of persons and places have been removed. In many places, words and phrases have been left in Hindi to capture their cultural specificity and complexity.

Analysis incorporated data immersion, data reduction and identification of common themes (Askham et al. 2007). Field diaries were read multiple times, before being typed and coded into broader categories and then compared with the interview data sets for repetition and comparison, similarities and differences using inductive methods (Markovic 2006; Ryan and Bernard 2003).

Codes were identified using techniques of repetition, indigenous typologies, metaphors, transitions, missing data and theory related material (Olszewski, Macey and Lindstrom 2006). From this, common themes began to emerge that were then subdivided where necessary (e.g., one subset of the 'Diagnosis' theme comprised 'tests' + 'theories of cause'). Meta themes were created by relating data sets with cohorts or settings (e.g., 'tests' + 'KSP'; 'tests' + 'hospital'+ 'families') and re-examined in relation to the peer reviewed literature. Such techniques ensured the rigour and validity of the data analysis.

Such a technical, mechanistic approach to categorize data has (hopefully) not been brought to bear on the quality of the writing. Rather the philosophy underpinning representation has been 'Can you (the reader) smell the writing?' A hermeneutic line of inquiry has been pursued to understand the dialectic between care practices and the discourses that frame them. Caregiving and care receiving are complex processes that are determined by cultural, economic and political scripts. People draw on these scripts in their everyday lives to interpret their realities and act accordingly. In the book, I seek to explain such interpretations as historically situated and practically oriented. Thus an interpretative social science has been followed (Rabinow and Sullivan 1987).

Limitations

I do not consider the challenges outlined earlier – being confused for a doctor, interruptions during the interviews and techniques of obtaining informed consent – to be limitations of the study. To my mind they represent the unique features of conducting interviews in India and are alternate ways that mature, adult relations can be built and respect accrued. Such challenges are not hindrances to the validity or reliability of the data. In such settings adherence to a textbook pro forma of how an interview should be done would belie the fundamental points of an interview – to *listen* to what people have to say and to how they say it. Rigidity does not ensure the rigour of data; it only guarantees that while some mythical auditor's checklist is ticked off somewhere, the people who participate in the study are less likely to consider participating again.

Nevertheless, there were some issues where my choice of ethnographic approach created theoretical 'blind spots' in my data and analysis. Moreover, the nature of my interviews did influence the kinds of questions that could be asked. For example, I never asked about sex. There is a dearth of work on the subject of dementia and sex anywhere and limited work on sexuality and ageing, under any circumstances, in India. Sarah Lamb's (2000) work shows that with age, there are somatic and sexual changes in identity. Women are meant to move from the 'heat' and 'openness' of the reproductive phase of their lives to a cooler, dryer post-reproductive life. Sexual energy is to be transformed into creative heat or *tāpas*, which can then be channelled into potent blessings and/or curses (van der Veer 1989). Such changes are not gender specific; men are also meant to be sexually 'cooler' and more disengaged from everyday life in old age. Becoming 'cooler' and celibate marks the elder's right to receive *sevā* and ability to give *pra-ṇām* (blessings). Diet is implicit within this paradigm and increased simplicity and plainness of food is believed to control sexuality and enhance asceticism.

However, in practice people do not always adhere to this blueprint for ageing. The more immediate needs of illness and intimacy may take precedence. Does sexual intercourse gradually stop because a spouse has dementia? How do marital relations change when demands for sex are increasingly made by the person with dementia? What if someone other than a spouse is propositioned? What are the alternate ways of enjoying intimacy? Such questions are not voyeuristic, but highlight points of transformation in caregiving relationships between spouses.

Families may also experience embarrassment because of inappropriate sexual behaviours and although no family ever broached the topic with me, according to Paul Issacs, a neurologist I interviewed in Kerala, sexually inappropriate behaviour was far more common than was admitted. Yet even he, with years of experience, could only recall one case where a family arrived in great distress because the seventy-five-year-old father with dementia was exposing himself to all the young women in the community. Sex and sexuality were rarely discussed by my participants and I could not ask about these deeply sensitive issues. They were inappropriate both because of the repeat interruptions and nature of the interviews and because of my youth and gender in a relatively conservative city. The closest I got to talking about sex was in conversations around food, sugar and love. Even here, discussions were allegorical, inferences at best.

Another limitation to this study is that no poor families caring for a person with dementia were part of the sample. As explained earlier, the sample was middle class and elite. The recruitment method, via ARDSI-DC, resulted in my coming into contact with few poor families. I tried to branch out and spent time in the government hospital OPDs to get a few more referrals from low-income families, but I had little success. I visited a district mental health clinic but the doctor was overworked and busy dispensing medications to a long line of people with schizophrenia and depression. No people with Alzheimer's were there either.

I also visited two slums on multiple occasions and consulted the community health services serving these neighbourhoods. But these services focused on maternal and child health, immunizations and capacity building; the community nurses could tell me how many abortions, pregnancies and babies each woman had, but the old were not in their ambit. When I began to query the women in the slum, many described circuits of migration; older people returned to their village while younger members migrated to the city. A few younger members would remain in the village to care for these older members and do *sevā* for them. Every three months or so, women would migrate to and from the village to work in the city and to care for children and the older middle-class Indians in their homes. If I 'really' wanted to talk to poor older people who might have dementia, I'd have to head into the rural interiors. But by this point it was April, I had been in India for four months and I had already found my interlocutors. I decided that this was a research topic for another day. I have included material on attendants and domestic servants and have tried to broaden the analysis on class by referring to the peer reviewed literature and my general observations. But such representations are one-sided and there are no voices of poor families caring for a person with dementia.

Additionally, because the sample was middle class and elite, nearly all the families I worked with had appropriated clinical terms such as 'dementia' and 'Alzheimer's'. On the one hand, this restricted work on local idioms of distress; on the other, it provided deeper insight into how the clinical category 'dementia' was folded into local understandings of illness and care. I describe this process in the following chapter and in work published elsewhere (Brijnath and Manderson 2011).

I also learned that despite being served by ARDSI-DC, many families had not absorbed the ideologies and vocabularies of the organization. As mentioned earlier, the Delhi Chapter's service delivery at the time was ad hoc and relied on volunteers' time and intermittent funding. Thus for most families the care experience tended to be a solitary one without strong support from ARDSI-DC. I did toy with the idea of diversifying my sampling strategy beyond ARDSI-DC but the richness of the information I was gathering, in combination with the desire to appease my university ethics committee and ensure there were some safety nets in place, resulted in the sample I obtained. Arguably, a different sampling strategy might have revealed another picture of dementia and locality in Delhi and urban India; perhaps a more 'shadowy' side where my enthusiasm and love for my project might have been eroded with exposure to those who did not want to care, who abandoned their relatives with dementia, where families fractured and broke and an altogether harder, more pitiless picture emerged. One can endlessly conjecture; however there are enough linkages between my findings and the existing literature for me to confidently state that this book offers an accurate (if incomplete) insight into what it is like for a middle-class family to care for a relative with dementia in urban India.

Finally, I wish that I had been able to pursue in greater detail logics and practices around transcendental medicine. I wanted to visit the practitioners that my participants had seen, but many had moved, stopped practising or were located in other cities. I did talk to an interlocutor who was familiar with the practices of Islamic transcendental healers but was not a healer himself. I unsuccessfully tried to persuade a community development worker from a local NGO in Nizamuddin to take me to the *dargāh*[7] and introduce me to various healers and I harassed a friend to take me to another site in Delhi where another pocket of transcendental healers were rumoured to be. I had no luck with either person. I eventually visited the Nizamuddin *dargāh* myself, only to joyously learn about the *qawwālī*;[8] I returned many times over the year to hear these songsters. But I never saw the transcendental healers; most likely I did not know what I was looking for or at. Eventually I realized that I could either focus on dementia care, within the limitations of the biomedical paradigm, or, like Alice wandering down a rabbit hole, spend my days in search of the exotic at the expense of what was right under my nose. I chose the former. But there is a lot to be said about transcendental medicine alongside the motivations which prompt anthropologists to go off in search of them.

In the following pages, biomedicine is privileged. So is the middle class and there is silence about sex. I have tried to counter these limitations with greater attention to class politics, discussions around love and relationality and by situating biomedicine within the social and cultural context of Delhi and India. I have tried to be evocative, analytical and emotive in my writing. I want you, the reader, to come away moved but also feeling uncertain, unsure about India. There are no easy answers. In short, I want you to smell the writing.

Notes

1. Some of the markers of difference between wealthy and poor suburbs include density of living (there are bungalows in richer suburbs; apartment blocks squashed together in poorer ones), the size and state of the roads (wide, smooth roads versus crumbling roads with potholes) and the supply of services like gas, water and electricity (poorer areas will get considerably less than wealthier ones).
2. Unfortunately, at the time of final editing (December 2013), more recent data on the age breakdown of Delhi's population were not available. The most recent published data were collected by the National Sample Survey Organisation in 2004.
3. These figures contrast markedly with the living arrangements of older people in the US where nearly 85 per cent of non-institutionalized older people live either only with their spouse or alone (US Administration on Aging 2013).
4. Kitty parties are women-only social gatherings typically held on weekdays during the daytime. They are usually attended by middle-class, wealthy housewives either in individuals' homes or at a public venue (e.g., restaurant). Kitty parties are notorious in Delhi for being gossipy and materialistic.
5. When British India was partitioned in 1947 into India and Pakistan, approximately 14.5 million Hindus, Muslims and Sikhs crossed these newly drawn borders to where they felt they constituted the religious majority. Muslims went to Pakistan, Hindus and Sikhs to India. Delhi received the largest number of refugees for a single city; its population increased by almost a million from 1947 (917,939 people) to 1951 (1,744,072 people) (Butalia 2002).
6. Dewing's (2007) method for interviewing people with dementia is as follows: background and preparation, establishing the basis for consent, initial consent, ongoing consent monitoring and feedback and support.
7. A *dargāh* is a shrine where a saint is buried and is a site of worship. The Nizamuddin *dargāh* is where the renowned Sufi saint Nizamuddin Auliya is buried. Also located here are the tombs of Amir Khusro (Sufi mystic) and Jehan Ara Begum (princess) and nearby is the tomb of Inayat Khan (Sufi mystic).
8. *Qawwālī* is a 700-year-old form of devotional Sufi music popular throughout South Asia.

2. THE DIAGNOSTIC PROCESS

My eldest daughter's father-in-law died and we all went [for the funeral] but he [Omar] wouldn't sit there. He was anxious about something. He would keep sitting down and standing up. From everything we could see, something was not right in his mind, something had become spoiled.

[Then] He went to Saudi [Arabia] for the Haj and when he came back, we could see from his eyes that something was troubling his mind. His mind wasn't working properly. He would confuse 1 lakh and 10 lakhs;[1] he would sometimes say the right thing and sometimes say the wrong thing. He would wear his clothes either inside out or the wrong way round. In the beginning this was happening. Then at one time I had some land that had to be sold and he experienced tension over this matter. 'Bring the money', he said, which he had never said before. 'Get the money from your mother and bring it. You've sold the land, now get your share and bring it to me'. We wondered what had happened to him because my family were his relatives as well. I said, 'Look at the way you're talking to your family. This is not the way', and I realized that there was something troubling him in his mind.

[So] we showed him to the neuro. Because what was happening was he would go out, he would travel all over Delhi but forget the way, he would drink a glass of water and forget that he had drunk it. We experienced a lot of problems at that time. And he would walk in the middle of the road, not on the side and Delhi is such a city that we would feel scared to send him alone. From these things, we felt that he was in some difficulty. So we showed him in the hospital. They did all the tests, it took a lot of time, we were in the line and we thought it's better to show him in one day. They saw him and said, 'He's not hurt, he's not in any pain, he has this kind of illness – Alzheimer's – and it is the kind of illness, which is not going to get better. There is no medicine for this'.

At that point, wherever anyone would say, we would show him there. We showed him here, we showed him there, there was no place we left or where we did not show him. We showed him in Apollo [hospital], in Ram Manohar

[Lohia hospital], in Pant [hospital], in Safdarjung [hospital], everywhere we showed him. But they all said the same thing. No one said that he was going to get better. That was it (*Shafia Khan, 54*).

He is 56. It's four years since it has been diagnosed but it's been much more. I think it's been about 6 years since the symptoms started manifesting themselves. So [he was] 49, late 49, when I realized that things were just not right. He became very argumentative. You see suddenly from a very rational person, any inconsequential topic he would pick up, [and] would turn into almost a vicious argument. And if I happened to be at fault, then it might turn into something physically violent which was very unlike him. I thought that my marriage was going to seed. It was frightening. And every time it used to happen, I used to cry fiercely and think, what is happening? Is he beginning to dislike me? What has gone wrong?

Then my daughter had this terrible problem [brain injury which required surgery] and we went to Trivandrum and he just didn't help me. He just receded into the background and there I had to explain everything to the doctor. And I was telling the doctor, 'Doctor, he is not himself' and out of the blue, the doctor said, 'Why don't you see a neurosurgeon?' I didn't realize what he was getting at because I was telling him the symptoms and he said, 'Just go to this doctor and he'll check'. And I went to Dr. Iyer who was supposed to be a specialist in dementia and they asked him questions and said, 'We'll just do these tests. We'll do a SPECT scan which hones into the area which is impaired'. And lo and behold, they discovered that he had the symptoms of dementia (*Josie Dharam Singh, 52*).

SHAFIA KHAN AND JOSIE DHARAM Singh live in south Delhi. They are women in their fifties, caring for their husbands, who are in the late stages of Alzheimer's disease. At the time of writing, Josie has already lost her husband; 'Su' (shortened from Surinder) has died. In all likelihood, Shafia is now a widow too. Both struggled to care for their husbands and will now struggle with widowhood and a new way of living at midlife. They have both lived with Alzheimer's disease and sickness, managing not only their husbands, their families and themselves, but accomplishing the financial callisthenics necessary for caring on a shopkeeper and school teacher's salary respectively.

There are many parallels in Shafia's and Josie's lives – marriage, children, illness, caring, widowhood and the genteel poverty of middle-class families on meagre wages. But there are also many differences: Shafia is a still and contained woman, her voice even and resolute; she is Muslim, from a small town in Uttar Pradesh, who had an arranged marriage to a member of her extended family with whom she had five children. She is of limited means but has pragmatically channelled her sewing talents into a little shop opposite her house, where she stitches 'suit pieces' for local women in her neighbourhood. Josie is a musician. She teaches piano at school and in private tuition and plays in the Church choir where she devoutly goes every Sunday evening to reaffirm her faith. Her voice is like her piano; it can be sharp or flat as it lilts and flows. She is a spritely woman, leaping to tend to things, most especially her beloved Su, her Sikh husband, with whom she had a love marriage and two children. Josie – Josephine – is originally from Andhra Pradesh in south India and has little family in Delhi. Her parents are dead, her sister lives overseas and her children are grown, married and live elsewhere. Her in-laws, who live in Delhi, have not really given her strong support.

Neither woman has met the other, nor, with the exception of Alzheimer's disease, would they have much to talk about if they did. Josie can be broadly located as upper middle class and Shafia would be classified as lower middle class. This is a question of capital and identity where gender, class and religion 'converge and produce instances of contestation and ambivalence' (Fernandes 2006: 166). Shafia lives in a neighbourhood where there have been police 'encounters' (shoot outs) with alleged terrorists. Josie lives about 3km away, in an area where security guards sit in front of individual houses to prevent 'encounters' with miscreants.

Women such as Josie and Shafia illustrate that Alzheimer's disease is not stratified by class, religion and socio-economic status. It afflicts people irrespective of their professional and moral careers and is often not diagnosed until the second stage when behavioural symptoms become more prominent and carers are less able to ignore the social disruptions these produce. Yet early diagnosis is critical for better management of dementia. Finances and care plans (including palliative care) can be organized and with medication and therapies, a certain quality of life can be preserved (Alzheimer's Australia 2007; Brodaty 2005). 'No time to lose!', the former slogan for Alzheimer's Disease International (2009), picks up on the importance of greater public awareness of dementia, early diagnosis and optimal care, improved access to healthcare services and of the rights of people living with dementia and those of their carers and families.

In this chapter I focus on how and why dementia diagnoses are typically made in the second stage of the disease. I argue that there are familial and patient barriers to early diagnosis because the symptoms are initially conceived as the cultural idiosyncrasies of old age and that there is a heuristic process whereby these 'normal' symptoms of ageing get translated into Alzheimer's disease. Diagnosis is not a straightforward process but occurs with time and in stages. This usually begins with a crisis leading to presentation at the clinic. Physiological and psychological tests follow, the diagnosis is determined based on these test results and the family is informed. Violence and resistance from the family to such news are typically the initial responses. Acceptance of the disease is gradual, as are families' explanations as to why this happened to their relative. I use three variations of the Hindi word '*dekh*' (see) – *dekhnā:* (to see), *dekhānā:* (to show) and *dikhnā:* (to be seen) – to describe how families experience this diagnostic journey, from the initial onset of the symptoms of dementia to the ultimate acceptance of a diagnosis.

देखना – *Dekhnā*: To See

In 2008, the *Diagnostic and Statistical Manual Version IV* (DSM-IV) (APA 2000) was the global psychiatric reference used to classify and diagnose all mental disorders, including various dementias and other neurocognitive disorders.[2] According to DSM-IV, an early indicator and key diagnostic feature of dementia was memory impairment. Memory impairment, when coupled with either aphasia, apraxia, agnosia and/or diminished higher executive functioning, could be diagnosed as dementia. These clinical features had to manifest over a period of time, significantly impact on social functioning and constitute a decline from the earlier capabilities of the patient. Refinements then follow to categorize the dementia into its subtypes such as Alzheimer's disease, vascular dementia or multi-infarct dementia, via a battery of neuropsychological, laboratory and other tests (APA 2000).

But at the same time, as outlined in the introduction, memory loss, cognitive and functional decline are seen in India (and elsewhere in Asia) as the normal social markers of ageing. Ageing and becoming *būṛhā* are the basis for the receipt of *sevā* by older people from younger family members. Consequently in many families with a relative with dementia, the initial symptoms were ignored in part because they were seen to be part of normal ageing and because of the care scripts governing *sevā* (e.g., younger women cook for older people; sons might do their parent's bank work).

In Shafia's and Josie's cases, early symptoms were perceived as socially disruptive but were not seen to have a pathological basis. Josie initially believed her marriage was 'going to seed'. She thought Su's gradual withdrawal, increased argumentativeness and violence were indicative of something having gone wrong with *her*. She only realized the problem lay in him, not her, when they went to Trivandrum for their daughter's brain surgery. On that trip, Josie suspected that something was medically wrong with Su because he packed only three of each personal item (three shirts, three trousers, three pairs of socks etc.) even though they planned to be away for some weeks. Compounding this, he was reticent to talk to the doctor, which Josie found incongruous, given his dominant role as an officer in the army and prior decisive behaviour in their marriage.

Other families had similar experiences of early symptoms, either ignored or interpreted as a normal part of ageing until there was some kind of 'crisis' or event that necessitated a visit to the doctor. Nandini described how she recognized things were not right and when she decided to take her father to a doctor:

> He had picked a lot of fights in the neighbourhood so they were all very anti him and he was being very aggressive. Secondly, things like personal hygiene; he was a person who even in the severest winter will have an ice cold water bath twice a day. I could see that it wasn't [happening]. And he wasn't concerned that I have come from far [to visit him]. Normally he is like, 'Have you had your breakfast?' These were small, small things but I could see that they weren't getting well ... And one thing – one of the neighbours stopped me during that visit and said, 'We'd like to know what your phone numbers are. Your father's been disturbing us a lot and we're thinking of hospitalising [him] and calling you'.

The neighbour's threat to Nandini, whether real or faked, served to reinforce her caring responsibilities. The threat implied that she had not been a 'good' daughter because she lived in another city to her father and that she needed to be embarrassed into fulfilling her responsibilities as a good daughter. Threatening to hospitalize her father also invoked the stigma associated with institutionalization. In the diagnostic context, a threat such as this prompted Nandini to reinterpret social misdemeanours as biological distress. For families, there were three events which created this transformation: (1) a crisis of relocation; (2) a medical crisis relating to another health condition; and (3) an emotional crisis. These typologies are artificial in their separation. Families typically experienced all three to varying degrees and these were grounds for medical intervention.

Crisis of Relocation

Relocation was physical and/or psychological and either shifted the responsibility of care to another family member or reaffirmed an existing family member's responsibility for caring. Symptoms became disruptive to a point where they could no longer be ignored or contained. For example, Parvati Gowda (43) took responsibility for her mother – Meenakshi (78) – moving her from Kerala to Delhi, because her mother could no longer keep account of her daily spending or manage the household budget. Parvati said, 'She was not having any [idea about] how much she was giving and what she had. That's when we thought that she needs full time care, so we brought her here'. In this case, physical relocation was also influenced by psychological fears around Meenakshi's isolation. Meenakshi's husband had passed away many years ago and after this, Parvati took on greater responsibility for caring for her mother. Spouses play a critical role in caring and covering for each other. Children, with the presence of both parents, tend to assume a secondary role and only really take on full responsibility when one parent has died or is incapable of providing care.

Money was a common reason for relocating or reaffirming care in parent-child and spousal relationships. Exigency centred on safeguarding financial security as families worried about how the person with dementia was handling everyday finances or vice versa. When Shafia sold her land, Omar's reaction to her obtaining her share of the money and bringing it to him, was the culmination of a series of unusual behaviours on his part. Disruptive behaviours, like forgetting the way home and wearing one's clothes inside out, could be downplayed, but Omar's confusion over money signalled that Shafia had to intercede and take him to the neurologist. In this case, financial responsibility from husband to wife was transferred via a medical diagnosis.

Concerns about safeguarding financial security point to wider anxieties around money, deception, family and class in India. Popular culture often draws on the negative imagery of children stealing property, frittering away hard earned resources and then denying care and *sevā* to older parents. There is a kernel of truth to this image: of the 518 murders registered in Delhi in 2008, the motives for 9 per cent of them were family disputes and a further 11 per cent were over property and money matters (Patnaik 2009). According to Inspector Tyagi in the Delhi Police's Senior Citizen Cell, over 50 per cent of the Cell's complaints came from lower middle-class older people and were about civil matters. The bulk of these complaints were about denial of food, not being served on time, pressure to sell the family property or to sign over the property. 'There is not much we can do', said Tyagi, 'but we always advise them to *never* sign property over, to always keep it in their control because the moment they do, the children stop caring. They won't do anything for them then'.

Medical Crisis for another Health Condition

In this category, the diagnosis of dementia occurred because of a pre-existing health condition or sudden injury. The family and the person with dementia were already involved in the healthcare system, often with either a psychiatrist or neurologist. Examples include situations such as Josie's. The surgery required for her daughter brought the family into the clinical purview of specialists such as neurologists, psychiatrists, neurosurgeons and the like. Su's retreat into the background caused Josie to grumble, 'Doctor, he is not himself'. Clinical presentation and diagnosis were opportunistic and tangential, as another health condition – in this case, their daughter's surgery – took precedence over the diagnosis.

Medical crises could also be unexpected. Consider Govind Ballabh Tandon (58) and his wife Sheila (58). Her diagnosis occurred after she suffered a head injury from a road accident on her way to work. Tandon recalled that following the accident, Sheila's temperament changed and 'she used to repeat the same thing. She took time to follow actions [instructions]'. Having interacted with doctors because of Sheila's accident, biomedicine provided the most immediate framework to interpret her behaviour. This made it the first avenue her family sought.

Emotional Crisis

In this category, the person to be diagnosed with dementia experienced a level of shock and/or depression. Often this shock resulted from the death of a loved one. No one had discerned K.P. Aggarwal's (69) symptoms of dementia, even though he was ailing for many years. After his father died, K.P'.s wife, Sita (63), recalls, 'He became so quiet'. K.P'.s silence was readily accepted by his family until he developed a problem with his balance. According to Sita, 'Something went wrong in his walking, he walked like an alcoholic. Everyone thought he was drinking' and so to avoid community censorship, the family took him to the doctor.

Nayantara's mother, Mrs Hamdari, on the other hand, was only taken to the doctor after a prolonged period of grief, which showed no signs of diminishing in its intensity. Mrs Hamdari (80) had watched her younger sister die a painful death and wept every day for over a year. According to Nayantara, 'Every morning when the maid used to come that was the story, '*Nani-ma* is crying' – she was crying all the time. I think, from what I remember, from the hospital cards, a year later I took her to the doctor'.

In these two cases, grief, whether quiet or noisy, was only reinterpreted as a medical symptom because it exceeded the culturally appropriate time to grieve and had a disruptive effect on the household. Mrs Hamdari's constant weeping and K.P'.s stumbling, over an extended period of time, attracted attention and commentary from outsiders like the maid, neighbours, relatives and friends. With no signs of healing or closure, K.P'.s and Mrs Hamdari's continuous bereavements or 'shocks' prompted their families to seek medical advice.

Through all these crises – relocation, medical intervention for another health condition, emotional trauma – families began to 'see' that something was not right. 'Seeing' was accumulative in that families saw numerous oddities that they were able to compile, post-diagnosis, into the symptoms of the 'disease' dementia. Pre-diagnosis, families were unaware of the pathology, prognosis and implications for care. What they would have seen would have increased their fears of the unknown and the additional responsibilities they would have to shoulder. As long as the symptoms of the dementia were viewed as part of *buddhāpan* for which *sevā* was to be provided, families operated within a social framework, which allowed for contestation and conflict. Without a formal diagnosis, the dementing person could behave irrationally and aggressively, argue over money, weep or be violent. Even so, some people with dementia identified that something was not right in themselves:

> In the initial stages she would cover up. She would say, 'There is nothing wrong with me, I'm 76 years old, I'm doing pretty well for someone who is 76'. But then one day she told me, '*Char deno ke ćāṅdnī pher andherī rat*' [four days of light and then it's night again] *(Namita Sood, 53)*.

> Initially I thought he was joking that he couldn't remember and that nothing was there. But he would just sit around and look at the TV and wouldn't interact with anyone so I thought, 'What's this?' *(Nina Bhagat, 70)*.

दिखाना – *Dekhānā*: To Show

Families often followed two pathways to the neurologist's door – either through direct consultation, or, rarely, through referral from a local doctor who recognized the broad brushstrokes of a neurological impairment. There were only around six to seven neurologists in Delhi who were qualified and willing to diagnose and manage people who had dementia. Those in the private sector largely shunned this task despite the chronicity of irreversible dementias, because the lack of a cure and concomitant degeneration reduced profit margins. Though this contradicts the common sense logic of long-term care equalling a steady income for doctors, Dr Bose, a geriatrician in a public hospital explained:

> After a while it becomes very difficult to ask for money from the patients. If they [practitioner] have seen someone three times or four times it becomes very difficult to ask for money on the fifth, sixth, seventh or twentieth time. After all it is very embarrassing for the practitioner and [there] is some amount of pain and shame. You can't be a vulture . . . you have to have some feelings. So there's not much business in it.

In the public health sector, ARDSI-DC had linkages with two government hospitals, where designated Out Patient Departments (OPDs) also functioned as 'memory clinics'. If a dementia diagnosis was made in these clinics, the neurologists, also members of ARDSI-DC's Governing Board, would refer the families to the NGO. In the rare event that the family came to ARDSI-DC prior to obtaining a diagnosis, the NGO would send them to the memory clinic to get a confirmed diagnosis. As a matter of course, the NGO made appointments for families in these OPDs. Typically appointments are not made in OPDs and people are seen on a first-come first-served basis. In theory, this was a strategy whereby families would not have to wait before seeing a doctor.

The Central Government of India has been running these two government hospitals since the 1950s. Both are teaching hospitals that offer general and specialist services such as cardiothoracic surgery, neuroscience, ophthalmology, emergency care and paediatrics. The doctors are knowledgeable and skilled; most senior registrars and consultants have a clinical research profile and have published in prestigious international and domestic medical journals. Many have worked in rural and urban India as well as overseas. As staff in a public hospital, their services and consultations are offered at little to no cost, so the poor and marginalized arrive in their millions each year. In the OPDs where I did my observations, between 1.2 and 1.5 million patients are treated each year. The doctors I directly observed, in an average OPD session of two hours, would see between 50 and 150 patients.

In OPDs, people waited for hours in uninviting halls on hard metal chairs. The chairs were black, in rows and under harsh fluorescent lights. People waited without complaint to be seen for two minutes by a doctor. Poor and lower middle-class people wore their best clothes – polyesters and synthetics of brassy pinks, greens, blue, grey, black and white. Wealthier people preferred private services and tended not to visit these hospitals; when they did, they wore the faded cottons, linens and denims of bourgeois understatement. Doctors conventionally wore white lab coats, pharmaceutical representatives wore expensive cologne and grubby anthropologists wore comfortable sandals. These hospitals were noisy, crowded, frenetic places. The basic equipment was meagre, the buildings worn; the staff were short of time and tempers ran high. There was no air conditioning or heating; only the proverbial dust.

The process of diagnosis within the government hospital setting was arduous and time-consuming. There were a series of tests to be administered, which commenced with a detailed case-history and neuropsychological tests that examined the cognitive features of memory, praxis, visio-spatial capacity, planning, judgement and money handling. Scales such as the Mini Mental State Exam (MMSE) were readily used in these settings. This is problematic because, as I have discussed elsewhere (Brijnath 2011a, 2011b), cultural and systemic factors affect score results and call into question the methods used to screen for dementia (see Iype et al. 2006; Mathuranath et al. 2005).

Following neuropsychological tests, there was a detailed medical history for stroke, hypertension, thyroidism and seizures; then followed an assessment of risk factors such as alcohol and smoking, an evaluation of the patient's diet (whether they were vegetarian or not), a complete blood count to rule out liver and renal diseases and finally, neuroimaging. These tests required the input of neurologists, psychologists, laboratory technicians, radiologists, nurses, ward staff and administrators. Seamless transitions from one test to the next were rare. Some patients were able to stay in the hospital, during which time the entire gamut of tests were run, but those families who lived in Delhi were often encouraged to come and go as per the appointment times they managed to schedule. This was perceived as less stressful on individual families and hospital resources. But long hours were spent waiting for doctors, tests and hospital administrative services – a well-documented complaint across nearly every public hospital in India (Mukhophadhyay 1989; Peters 2002; Purohit 2004). Many families, like Shafia's, made the strategic decision, based on factors such as the health of their loved one or time away from work, to try and complete all the tests in one exhausting day, rather than over a period of time. Often this time period, whether over one day or one week, was when the clinician spent the most (sometimes the only) time with the person experiencing dementia. Although a follow up with the patient was meant to happen every three to six months to trace the progress of their disease, the current symptoms, the need for drug management and provide counselling for the family, in practice this rarely occurred because of time constraints and patient numbers.

When asked, families spent little time describing the diagnostic process despite the challenges they faced. Instead, for them, neuroimaging was pivotal, especially the MRI (Magnetic Resonance Imaging). In contrast, doctors described the MRI as one of the least important and last tests that they administered, one done more to confirm, than to guide, their suspicions.[3] For families with whom I worked, neuroimaging served as a marker of the doctor's credibility and a signifier of good clinical knowledge and practice. Thirteen families explicitly mentioned the MRI and another three specifically named the SPECT (single photon emission computed tomography) scan when asked to describe the diagnostic process. As Josie said after Su's SPECT scan, 'Lo and behold they discovered that he had the symptoms of dementia'.

As the penultimate point in the diagnostic process, the MRI reflects the indigenization and appropriation of this particular biomedical technology within India. Appropriation as defined by Hahn (2004) and extended by

Granado and colleagues (2011) is syncretic and procedural. It involves the appropriation of an object or idea to begin, then its objectification within an established local dialectic, followed by the incorporative actions related to this new object or idea and finally its transformation that redefines it according to local customs and norms. Put simply, the appropriation of neuroimaging into local understandings was how the cultural stamp of approval was given to a clinical diagnosis. Having an MRI validated for families that their relative was receiving all the benefits of biomedicine, which in turn reinforced the notion that to be treated 'properly' was to have an MRI or other brain scans. Mark Nichter (2008, 2002) found that the process of obtaining a scan in India serves as an idiom of concern by families and an idiom of distress by patients. Similarly Van Hollen (2003) and Pinto (2004) found that particular pharmaceuticals (oxytocins) and technologies (injections) were bound in cultural discourses of power and legitimacy. In south India, women's demands to receive oxytocins to induce labour were linked to ideas of women's strength and their capacity to courageously suffer the pains of childbirth, as well as shorter labour and therefore truncated hospital stay (Van Hollen 2003). In north India, the ability to administer injections was how ersatz practitioners demonstrated technical ability, access to institutions and biomedical knowledge (Pinto 2004). Thus legitimacy and power are articulated through embodied exchange and meta conversations about who receives, versus who administers and interprets, particular technologies (Pinto 2004: 353).

For the families in my study, the MRI and the SPECT scans offered, literally, a direct insight into the mind of the person experiencing dementia. It did not matter that families could neither read these scans nor interpret the highly medicalized language in the accompanying reports. Simply obtaining the MRI or the SPECT became a critical step through which families began to convert social misbehaviours into a biological pathology, *buddhā-pan* into Alzheimer's disease, social knowledge into neurological illiteracy, the known into the unknown.

Integral to this process was the use of language; the doctor's capacity to be able to read the scan, to identify the 'dark spots', to translate the technicalities in the report and to distil it into simple language, became a means by which their authority and pronouncement of the diagnosis was validated. Language also played an important role in determining what families understood of these explanations. Often family members switched from Hindi into English and then back again during the course of their explanation, although the key words were always spoken in English. Chintu explained her mother-in-law's dementia thus: 'Cell-vell weak *hai*, cell damage *ho gaya: aur* weak *hai*' (her cells in her brain are weak . . . in some cases her cells are damaged and in others they are weak). Similarly

Mamta Aggarwal said: 'Brain *mei thoṛa:* shrink *hota: hai, sārā* body parts *kā:m karne bānd kar deta hai*' (there is a little shrinkage in the brain and all the body parts stop working).

Joseph Dumit (2004) in his analysis of brain scans in the US, argued that images such as MRIs are used to delineate 'normal' and 'abnormal' brains and formed the basis on which assertions about the biology of mental states can be made. When linked to the imagery of 'shrinking' and cell death in the brain, such scans created a trajectory of decline: cell weakness and damage led to eventual cell death and shrinking of the brain. The use of English words such as 'weakness', 'damage', 'cell death' and 'shrink' also became a method by which Alzheimer's disease and dementia were distinguished from its Hindi counterpart, *buddhāpan*. This process of conceiving dementia varied by gender and age; younger women, particularly daughter-in-laws, keenly absorbed whatever the doctor's explanation was and reproduced the words verbatim when I spoke to them. This appropriation of a clinical category is indicative of younger Indians' increasing exposure to and enthusiasm for new types of medications, therapeutic regimes, biomedical technologies and disease categories and is a far cry from the lament of modernity and 'bad' families from a decade ago (Brijnath and Manderson 2011). In contrast older family members did not dwell on the pathophysiology of a person with dementia; for them, the causes of the disease had social rather than neurological origins. These etiologies usually developed following the acceptance of the dementia diagnosis and I will return to their viewpoints later.

Delivering the Diagnosis and Prognosis

For twelve families, the delivery of the diagnosis was the first time they heard the words 'Alzheimer's' or 'dementia'. Doctors had the dilemma of deciding just how much of the prognosis to reveal. This is a universal concern for physicians with three factors affecting truth telling practices: (1) the anticipated harmful and beneficial consequences of the truth; (2) belief in the patient's rights and autonomy; and (3) the physician's sense of duty and responsibility (Vanderpool and Weiss 1987). In Western countries, where the culture of individualism dominates, terminal patients are always included in discussions about their diagnosis and prognosis. However in other settings, patients may sometimes be shielded from this information by their families and doctors. For doctors the focus is not on truth telling or ascertaining patient wants but on preventing distress and giving the patient hope (see Ghavamzadeh and Bahar 1997; Kaufert 1999; Malik and Qureshi 1997).

In my study, doctors often delivered their diagnosis and prognosis in one sitting, in settings defined by time pressures, competing patient demands, lack of privacy and strict medical hierarchies. Here the doctor was the main authoritative figure and the families were passive quiet recipients of this medical knowledge. Tandon describes how he was informed of his wife's dementia:

> We took her to the neurologist at the hospital. He told me that she has dementia, Alzheimer's. I was hearing these words for the first time. I didn't even know what dementia or Alzheimer's was. That was at the initial stage and I said, 'Let's see what the doctor has to say'. The doctor told me, 'This is a progressive disease, incurable and not curable'. That was the first thing he said to me. Then, 'You have to care for her, you have to do it' (*Govind Ballabh Tandon, 58*).

> They saw him and said, 'He's not hurt, he's not in any pain, he has this kind of illness – Alzheimer's – and it is the kind of an illness which is not going to get better. There is no medicine for this' (*Shafia Khan, 54*).

At this stage, there was little realization among families of the far reaching impact of the diagnosis. While there was an acknowledgement that life would change, the intensity and depth of these changes were only realized incrementally as the disease progressed. Little information was made available to families; often they were referred to ARDSI-DC where usually they were given a caregiver's handbook either in Hindi or English. Compiled by one of the neurologists affiliated to ARDSI-DC, the book details how the disease progresses, management strategies for challenging behaviour, activities of daily living and stimulation for people with dementia. Some found the wealth of information overwhelming: 'I didn't even finish the book, I just read like two pages and was really worried. I said, "I'm not reading anymore, I've got to show him to a doctor"' (*Suneeta Sadhwani, 41*).

Giving families pamphlets, books and other printed materials rather than face-to-face delivery of such information was common even in private medical practice. Sunil Bhatnagar, an eminent neurologist in private practice in Delhi, described how he delivered the diagnosis:

> There is a book which I give all the families. First I send the patient out because I genuinely believe that you never know how much your patient understands and how much your patient doesn't understand. Then early in the diagnosis I tell them [the family], 'Look, there is some concern about the memory issues and that is why you have come to me'. I am very well known. [Then I say] 'We're not going to make the diagnosis right now. Let me see him again in three to six months so then we know'. And then time tells, the family comes to know themselves. So you don't have to hit them on day one,

'Look, this is what the person has, it is Alzheimer's disease, thank you, now go away'.

Bhatnagar's approach differed from what occurred in *sarkari* (government) hospital settings and was more in line with the DSM-IV recommendations for tracking symptom development over time (APA 2000). But both he and the *sarkari* doctors tended to deliver the diagnosis to the family and not to the person experiencing the dementia. Such an approach to the communication of chronic or terminal illness diagnosis and prognosis fits within a broader South Asian setting wherein patients are shielded from such knowledge by their doctors and family in a bid to maintain their optimism and prevent them from losing hope (see Bennett 1999; Lang 1990; Li and Chou 1997). A study from neighbouring Pakistan, on physician truth telling in cancer, found that patients were usually not informed of their diagnosis, often at the family's request (see Malik and Qureshi 1997). Families feared such news would devastate the patient, worsen his/her quality of life and hasten death. Doctors, in turn, withheld discussing such information with the patient, citing reasons like strong family support (kin members could communicate such news), fear of miscommunicating or introducing misconceptions, feelings of frustration and despair in dealing with cancer and the effects of therapy (Malik and Qureshi 1997).

In Alzheimer's disease, the chronicity and degenerative nature of the condition influenced the treatment doctors prescribed, which was not medical management but a social mandate to care. How the prognosis was framed, the manner in which it was delivered and the environment in which it was delivered affected families' receptiveness to this information. Even those who had heard of Alzheimer's disease and dementia struggled to accept the implications of diagnosis-care *fait accompli*. In five cases, the diagnosis itself was initially rejected.

Disappointment with the news of the diagnosis, combined with the family's experiential knowledge of the *sarkari* hospitals, resulted in feelings of disappointment in the doctor and many sought alternative diagnoses elsewhere. Such feelings are commonplace, especially in the mental health sector, as demonstrated in studies done on depression and schizophrenia in south India (Raguram et al. 2001; Saravanan et al. 2007).

दिखना – *Dikhnā*: To Be Seen

Disappointment, denial and resistance in relation to the diagnosis often led to doctor shopping. Doctor shopping includes the practice of people seeking multiple clinical opinions for the same health complaint; here I use the term specifically to refer to the practice of obtaining second (and third) opinions from allopathic doctors. 'Doctor shopping' is typically deployed pejoratively in the West, referring to prescription drug seeking behaviour (Hall et al. 2008; Martyres, Clode and Burns 2004). In India, doctor shopping is part of a pluralist, albeit hierarchical, healthcare system and has a historical basis; this will be detailed in the following chapter. In the Asian theatre, doctor shopping has been linked to chronicity (if the illness is recurring and/or progressive), the inability of patients to understand the doctor's explanations and scepticism about the doctor and the treatment plan (Hagihara et al. 2005; Sato et al. 1995). When families decided to switch doctors they reiterated these findings:

> He [the doctor] didn't have anything to communicate. He would act like he knew everything and we just had to listen to his prescriptions and do what he told us (*Nayantara Sen, 58*).

> I went to the doctors and they said, 'It looks like he's not going to get well'. That was enough for me and then I met another doctor who told me, 'Oh ma'm, be prepared, the worst is yet to come'. So he told me the same thing. Then my son took him to Singapore and had him checked there also. And he [doctor] said, 'Oh yes, be prepared for the worst and how far it goes' (*Nina Bhagat, 70*).

There is a correlation between class and allopathic doctor shopping; studies from Hong Kong (Johnston et al. 2006) and New Zealand (Barnett and Kearns 1996) have found that poor people are less likely to engage in this practice while those who are willing to pay have a greater propensity to do so. Conversely in India, while people's ability to change allopathic doctors is influenced by their income and capacity to pay for services, it is also mediated by broader understandings of public and private services. Long queues and overcrowding in government hospitals for free medicines and consultations are balanced against the immediate availability and fees associated with the private practitioner. Decisions to utilize particular services are based on income, time, qualifications and professionalism of the practitioner and the kinds of medications dispensed (e.g., analgesics and antibiotics) (Das 2003; Van Hollen 2003).

Doctor shopping also has cultural roots in *sevā* and the sick role. Despite the fact that the diagnosis identified a defined illness, doctors were unable to offer hope of a cure and only a script to care. Many families resisted their new roles by desperately seeking a different outcome from another doctor. Also, through seeking different opinions, families were able to display publicly not only how desperate they were for a different diagnosis, but also how much *sevā* they undertook for their loved one. In the Khan's case, despite receiving a diagnosis from one hospital, Shafia and her children took Omar to 'show' him in a number of other public and private hospitals across Delhi. Given the family's limited financial resources, accessing services in a private hospital affected their savings but the money was nevertheless spent to show people outside the immediate family just how much they cared for Omar. Shafia said, 'Wherever anyone would say, we would show him. We showed him here, we showed him there, there was no place we left or where we did not show him'.

To show or to take a sick person to the doctor are public acts that draw on the emotional and material currency of *sevā*. In the Khan family, they were able to show their extended family and friends how much *sevā* they were willing to do for Omar, by travelling all over Delhi with him. *Sevā* for Omar within their home was private, i.e., the onus rested on other people to come and see how much *sevā* they were doing, to validate that they were good carers and moral people. Taking him into the public arena to show him to a doctor, enabled more people to make this judgement swiftly. Yet this showmanship is temporary, because as the person begins to decline and doctors reiterate the same message of incurability, families are forced to accept the diagnosis. Shafia herself conceded, '[When] no one said that he was going to get better; that was it'.

Patients and Carers: Caring and Patience

In accepting the diagnosis, families began to resign themselves to their roles as 'carers'. This was not an easy process. Concomitant with resistance to the initial diagnosis and subsequent doctor shopping was violence and aggression. Feelings of frustration, confusion, denial of the disease and an inability to cope mounted as carers learnt through trial and error how to care. Although considered taboo, physical violence towards the person with dementia did occur in some families and as has been found in other settings, such violence was closely related to behavioural disturbances in the person with dementia, difficulties in communication and familial distress (Cooney, Howard and Lawlor 2006; Paveza et al. 1992).

Nina Bhagat, for example, admitted to hitting her husband, Karamjit, when he made *faux pas*, like coming out naked from the bathroom or not using the commode when he had to go to the toilet. Nina's violence was also underwritten by desperation to find an alternative to the narrative of decline. For her, accepting Karamjit's dementia meant conceding defeat and giving up:

> I felt it was wrong for them telling me to be prepared that he's going to be a cabbage in 10 years or he's going to be a cabbage in 15 years. I am not prepared to accept that. It is wrong. In 5 years or 15 years, whether we are cabbages or not, I will keep fighting. Whatever happens, will happen, there may be some deterioration but I still have hope and I still feel he will come back to me. I have not given up because mentally he is becoming more and more alert.

Thus even seven years after Karamjit's diagnosis Nina could not bring herself to accept his dementia. She felt her husband was 'pretending', the doctors were unduly pessimistic and a cure could be achieved. She made Karamjit undertake speech therapy, yoga, golf and reading and writing, in addition to giving him allopathic, *Āyurvedic* and herbal treatments. Through all these activities, Nina felt that Karamjit's brain could be re-activated and he would be fully functional again. When Karamjit resisted these activities or failed to complete them, Nina would become so angry she would also hit herself. She describes these *'maha'* (huge) fights:

> Even now when he doesn't listen, fighting comes automatically to me. He literally starts trembling when I get into this mood and then he holds me so tight that I can't breathe. He will tell me, 'No, no, you will not be this angry, you will not hit yourself'. I start hitting myself, I don't know what else to do. So he holds me so tight that I can't breathe [and says] 'No, No', till I calm down. Now each time we have a fight he holds me tight.

Not all carers were like Nina. For most, inflicting physical violence on the person with dementia was a major turning point in their struggle to accept the diagnosis. Nayantara described the initial period following her mother's diagnosis as 'terrible', because this was the time when she, her sister and her father struggled to come to terms with it. Her father, Mr Hamdari, was particularly aggressive as he struggled with managing his own high blood pressure which was exacerbated by the repetitive behaviours of his wife. Things changed after he hit his wife. He said, 'Finally, she hit me and I [holds up right hand] hit her back. This happened twice. Then I felt very guilty [pauses and then whispers], very guilty'.

Mr Hamdari's violence against his wife prompted his change in attitude. His remorse at his own actions induced greater acceptance of his wife's dementia and though his frustrations occasionally boiled over, he never hit his wife again. For most families, with acceptance came a reduction in violence on the carer's part and increased recognition of the diminishing capacity of the person with dementia.

When the scenario was reversed, i.e., when the person with dementia was violent or hostile, the behaviour was dismissed as the pathology of the disease not caused by social triggers. The tempo of the household was unaffected, even though there were instances of injury. Few sought respite by sending the person with dementia to another family member or to an institution.

Brain and the Social Body

With acceptance of the diagnosis came the beginnings of a social etiology of dementia. The old critique of urbanization, modernization, industrialization and westernization, all linked to dementia and Alzheimer's disease (see Cohen 1998), still echoed in some service delivery circles. Among families this etiology was linked to the pathophysiology of the disease and a broader lamentation about the vagaries of contemporary urban life. As mentioned, older family members did not talk about brains drying, shrinking, becoming weak or damaged. For them the disease had social rather than neurological origins.

Urban life, in Delhi, was defined by time, tension and loneliness – and all were underpinned by a complaint about the increasing tendency towards individualism. Having 'enough time' served as a measure of family members' ability and willingness to engage. Younger people, usually women, rarely seemed to have enough time, engaged as they were either in paid employment or the more laborious itineraries of housework and childcare (no matter the age of the children). Many primary carers (usually older women) accepted that lack of time was a justification for the tertiary roles that younger women assumed in caregiving. Sita described how her daughter helped her to care:

> If we have to go to the hospital then she'll send the car. If I am in any jam then she'll send the car. If there is any work she will do it. She helps me a lot. She calls almost every day and we talk. Or I'll call her. She doesn't come a lot, maybe once in 20–30 days [because] *she doesn't get time*. I was supposed to go today but it wasn't possible, so I'll go tomorrow. *She has a busy life and not much time* (emphasis added).

Related to a lack of time was an increase in tension or stress. 'Don't take tension', was frequently counselled in everyday conversation and directed to people who were seen to be 'taking tension' or experiencing high levels of stress. Too much tension was believed to lead to dementia, depression and psychosis, findings that have been made elsewhere in India (Parkar, Fernandes and Weiss 2003; Saravanan et al. 2007, 2008). Tandon linked his wife Sheila's dementia to time and tension:

> In city life everyone is busy. Everyone locks up their houses and goes off to work. There is a lot of tension in life – my two sons were working and I was busy with my business, I had to go outstation most of the time. Everyone had their own keys, came and went at their own time. Maybe this is one of the causes. Tension was present.

Implicit within this etiological paradigm was loneliness. 'Too much tension' when coupled with little time led to people feeling stressed and alone; this in turn, was seen to lead to dementia. Said Suneeta:

> Based on what I have seen within my own family, loneliness seems to be the biggest reason. My aunt's husband [had just] died when she started experiencing this problem. All her children were busy in their work, her grandchildren were busy in their work, there was no one for her to talk to.

Josie's children also felt that their father's illness was brought on by 'utter loneliness'. Josie recounted that she and Su spent most of their married lives apart as she cared for various ill family members and he served in the armed forces in various warzones. But she baulked at the idea of loneliness leading to dementia, based on her own experiences of being alone and self-reliant. In contrast she perceived Su had adequate social support while he was in the army (friends, camaraderie, team sports and social outings). Nevertheless, she accepted that Su's experience of being lonely may have been different from hers, just as Tandon accepted that Sheila 'took more tension' than he did when he recalled their working lives. At this level, carers adopted a phenomenological understanding of the lives of people living with dementia, i.e., they accepted that their loved one's social construction of the world was different to their own worldview and that their loved one's experiences of being alone could have led to their dementia.

Carers also sought to distinguish between themselves and the person with dementia. To begin, whether openly acknowledged or implicit, some deficiency in lifestyle and/or individual personality of the person with dementia was assumed, leaving them unable to cope with modern urban life and therefore vulnerable to the disease. Deficiency, however, was not blame, merely a platform through which carers could highlight their own strengths and benevolence in coping and caring. Carers did not equate deficiency with blame because it could also highlight their contributing roles in their social etiologies. Thus Tandon admitted that he worked too long and was away too much, not that this contributed to Sheila's loneliness. Josie conceded that Su might have been lonely but did not link it to her prolonged separation from him. There was delicate silence around such an obvious link.

Conclusions

Three types of 'seeing' have been used to describe how families experience the diagnostic journey, from the initial onset of the symptoms of dementia to the ultimate acceptance of a diagnosis: (1) *dekhnā:* (to see); (2) *dekhānā:* (to show); and (3) *dikhnā:* (to be seen).

Initially, families had 'to see' that something was wrong. They had to differentiate a medical pathology in a cultural category and separate dementia from *buddhāpan*. This was done through a compilation of strange behaviours, leading to crises and eventual clinical presentation. Then families had 'to show' their older relative to a doctor. Their experiences with neuroimaging played a key role in how they began to see the dementia and conceive of the illness. The MRI, in particular, was related to the linguistic and social separation of old age and Alzheimer's disease. Families' experiences were also shaped by institutional cultures and resource shortages in hospitals. This affected their level of acceptance towards the diagnosis and many resisted the idea that there was no cure and only long-term caring. This often prompted people into seeking solutions elsewhere; denial and doctor shopping were common. Doctor shopping was also linked to the public display of *sevā*, as some families sought 'to be seen' to be pursuing all avenues and being good carers.

With acceptance, social etiologies began to be developed. Families began to fold the biological into the social to develop an integrated framework that accommodated both neurological and social pathology. Daughters-in-law used English instead of Hindi to reproduce what they had understood from the doctor, whereas older spouses tended to resort to the discourses of tension, time and loneliness in modern Delhi life.

The diagnostic process became the signifier of upheaval in families' lives and marked the beginning of a road of caring for a person living with dementia. It left its influence in the long term, in how often families visited the doctor, complied with medicines, sought alternatives and which health system they ultimately put more faith in. I describe these treatment pathways in the following chapter.

Notes

1. As of 16 December 2013, 1 lakh= A$1,794.72; 10 lakh = A$17, 946.35
2. In June 2013, DSM-IV was superseded by DSM-V (APA 2013). In the new manual there were significant changes to the diagnostic criteria for dementias. First, the term 'dementia' was replaced by the term 'major neurocognitive disorders.' Key diagnostic features of major neurocognitive disorders include: (1) significant cogni-

tive decline in one or more cognitive domains: complex attention, executive function, learning and memory, language, perceptual-motor, or social cognition; (2) evidence that the severity of the decline is causing interference with independence in everyday activities; (3) evidence that the decline must not have occurred exclusively within the context of a delirium; and (4) evidence that the decline cannot be better explained by another mental disorder (e.g. major depressive disorder, schizophrenia).
3. An MRI scan is usually obtained to rule out other possible conditions (such as tumours and reversible dementias) and to supplement clinical diagnoses. It also allows better differentiation between mild cognitive impairment and Alzheimer's disease and enables tracking the development of the former to the latter (Knopman et al. 2001; Scheltens and Korf 2000).

3. THERAPEUTICS AND HEALTH SEEKING

I am following the science daily [and] any day now some treatment will come. It hasn't come till now but it will happen. Up until now no one cared about this disease – now everyone's energies are on it, so the treatment will emerge. It maybe that we don't get the benefit, that we're not capable but I keep hoping that we can, that in between something can happen . . . there is a lot of effort being made in medical science. God knows. This is my ultimate objective, I have no mission, no life, no earnings, this is it – that there is some treatment. I look at the website daily, I correspond daily, I keep looking, I keep researching . . . (*Govind Ballabh Tandon, 58*).

Mrs Sethi: *Iska ilāj hai kuch?* (Is there any *ilāj* for this?)
Nehi (no)
Koi ilāj nehi de sakta? (There is no *ilāj* that you can give us?)
Till now – I'm not a doctor and I can't give a 100 per cent guarantee – but till now in my research, in all that I have read, there isn't any.
Hamne vēsa chhora nehi Dilli mē, koyee ilāj nehi chhora (There is nowhere in Delhi that we have left, there is no *ilāj* that we haven't tried).

ILĀJ (PRONOUNCED E-LAAJ) MEANS 'CURE' and 'to treat medically' in Hindi, Urdu, Persian, Arabic and Turkish. It is frequently used and articulates a dream of regeneration against a backdrop of slow degeneration. Every family sought an *ilāj*. For some, like Tandon, it had become the 'ultimate objective' that defined their lives. The quest for an *ilāj* was also a search for hope and usually began during diagnosis, when families went doctor shopping in a bid to find an alternative to the narrative of chronicity, decline and long-term care that confronted them. Long after the diagnosis had been accepted, this search continued as behavioural symptoms of the disease and unrelated comorbidities (such as cataracts, diabetes or heart problems) rose and abated. To search for an *ilāj*, a powerful marker of *sevā*, reiterated the family's devotion and love for the person with dementia. Mrs Sethi said, 'There is nowhere in Delhi that we have left, there is no *ilāj* that we haven't tried'. For Mrs Sethi, *ilāj* was also a lament about the inability of health practitioners to provide any kind of a cure, merely an instruction to care. Her frustration stemmed from broader beliefs in the power of medicine to cure all ills, as she could not understand how such a powerful epistemology could offer no hope.

Biomedicine's capacity to offer a cure and/or improved medications has become the foundation of hope in dementia. Charities and NGOs press for donations to fund medical research and governments allocate considerable sums to medical researchers to come up with a vaccine or cure. Moreira and Palladino (2005) argue that biomedicine is shaped by two contrary temporal logics: 'regimes of hope' and 'regimes of truth'. 'Regimes of hope' are uncertain, risky and linked to new technologies. They are future oriented – the hope that a cure is in the 'pipeline'. 'Regimes of truth' are present oriented, premised on the existing evidence and past outcomes. To date neither cure nor effective medication has been achieved for dementia and death is inevitable. In a regime of truth, patients and families are positioned as consumers and autonomous agents in determining palliation. In a regime of hope, they are more desperate and risky, costly and closely monitored treatments are more likely to be sought. But truth and hope are unevenly juxtaposed in India; hope takes precedence over truth and is central to maintaining relations between the doctor, the patient and the patient's family.

This chapter examines how people perceive of an *ilāj*, persist in their search of one and the socio-political context of medical care in contemporary India. The power relations between doctors and patients and the immediate and gradual outcomes of these interactions, are critical to the search for an *ilāj*. In the trials and tribulations of everyday life in Delhi's public health system, *ilāj* is part of a biomedical montage that propagates the abuse of power through the normalization of bureaucratic hierarchies and insufficient resources. This will be explained by drawing on my observations in neurology OPDs and carers' reports of their experiences in government hospitals.

When families move from the hospital to the home, the power of *ilāj* – embodied in this journey as pharmaceutical drugs – reverberates in its physiological and relational effect. The physical and psychological side effects of these drugs heighten carer surveillance of the person with dementia. Families' experiences with pharmaceutical drugs influenced how often they visited clinical doctors, complied with medicines and sought traditional and transcendental healers. Ultimately, which health system they trusted was based on its outcomes for both the health of the person with dementia and the entire family.

I begin via a seemingly circuitous route – the etymology of *ilāj*. It is essential to understand the history of medical pluralism in India and the doctor-patient relationship within this context. This history will contextualize how class, gender, religion and education are deployed in contemporary experiential understandings of illness and care. It will also define the scope of terms such as 'health practitioners' (biomedical, traditional and transcendental), 'patient rights' in their past and current application and highlight the complexity of the challenges confronting Indian medical care today.

The Etymology of *Ilāj*

Ilāj is an Arabic word and its incorporation into Hindi underscores the cultural, linguistic and political fusion between the Middle East and India, of which medical pluralism is an offshoot. Even before the Arabs reached Indian shores in the seventh century, Indian medicine, within the boundaries of the subcontinent, was diversifying. *Āyurveda*[1] (*āyus* means longevity; *veda* is knowledge) was a complex epistemology that had absorbed the class stratifications of the post Vedic *Dharmashastra* texts,[2] the humanist ideologies of Buddhism and the inclusion of metals in its pharmacopeia (Bala 2007). Its permeability reflected its medico-pantheistic origins, which combined religion, magic, physiology, anatomy and pathology. The literary foundations of *Āyurveda* were articulated in the *Rgveda* and *Atharvaveda*, two of the four *Vedas*, and the earliest sources of medical literature in the world, in circulation from around 2500-2000 BC. *Āyurvedic* practices had an even earlier genesis in the third millennium BC in the ancient cities of Mohenjo-Daro and Harappa, where municipal sewage and drainage, public baths and the use of plants had both preventative and therapeutic value for health, as well as religious value (Bala 2007; Leslie 1969).

The arrival of the Arab traders in the seventh century heralded an exchange of medical knowledge and practices between India and the Levant. These cross pollinations were reflected in the writings of Islamic physicians from the tenth and eleventh centuries onwards and in the introduction into India of *Unani* medicine, itself a syncretism of Greek, Arabic, Persian, Indian and Chinese influences (*Yūnān* means 'of Ionia or Greek'). In 1279, with the Latin translation of Muhammad B. Zakariya Al-Razi's magnum opus *Kitab al-Djami 'al-kabir*, or 'Great Medical Compendium', elements of Indian medicine made it into the European clinic (Goodman 2009). In India, following the founding of the Mughal Empire in 1526, *Unani* medicine began to be organized into a discrete system which existed alongside *Āyurveda*. However, *Āyurveda* was the medicine for the masses and *Unani* was for the ruling class (Patterson 1987).

During this time, what is commonly now called 'folk' medicine was also practised. Folk medicine tends to comprise a set of sympathetic magico-religious practices, which include mantras, curses and miracles, typically practiced by *Gurus*, *Babas* and *Pīrs*[3] (amongst others) (Langford 2003). The term 'folk' is problematic in the Indian context, as it neither sufficiently captures the theological richness and complex practices of this kind of medicine, nor does it define the socio-political location of the various 'folk' who access it. Don Bates (1995) has argued that biomedical and traditional epistemologies stake their legitimacy in literary texts, medical textbooks and professional training, unlike faith healers who often rely on revelations and oral histories. This distinction is contestable in India as texts such as the Qur'an, the *Bhagavad-Gita* and the Bible contain moral precepts that transcendental medicine practitioners either draw on as *Gurus*, *Babas* and *Pīrs*, or set themselves in opposition to as *kala jādū* (black magic) practitioners. In addition, there are particular logics and practices that are common to particular healers, suggesting a level of 'professionalization' and training. When Muslim healers, for example, put a *tabeez*[4] in water and tell patients to drink that water over many days, until all the script has disappeared, the *ilāj* is imagined as one literally ingesting the word of God to ward off the effects of curses that had led to the presenting of either physical and/or psychological ills.

This type of medicine sits apart from traditional medicines (e.g., *Āyurveda*) and biomedicine and I use the more specific term 'transcendental medicine' to delineate it rather than 'folk' medicine. Such conscious use of terminology is indicative of the power plays that have, over time, resulted in a hierarchical (re)organization of biomedicine, traditional medicine and transcendental medicine in India. 'Biomedicine' deliberately replaces 'Galenic' medicine to reinforce its hegemony rather than its historical roots; 'traditional' has replaced 'indigenous' medicine to reinforce its chronicity and cross pollination rather than its nativity to India; and 'transcendental' replaces 'folk' to evoke the religiosity embedded within it.

Despite constant attempts at boundary marking, these three medicines have fluid alliances and bleed into each other. For example, transcendental medicine, which has had historical links to both traditional medicine in India (see Kakar 1991; Langford 2003) and biomedicine in Europe (see Porter 1997, 2002), also formed a bridge between these two in India. Early timorous ventures by the Europeans, first by the Portuguese in the sixteenth century and later by the English in the seventeenth century, mobilized religion in healthcare. British chaplains touted Hindu's abstinence from alcohol and meat, their high fibre diets and light dress as evidence of their piety. These dietary and lifestyle maxims are found in Hindu scriptures and in texts (Wujastyk 2003). The British chaplains' exhortations, however, were not driven by a quest for a higher morality, but by a search for lower mortality as the European diet of meat and copious amounts of alcohol and heavy ceremonial dress saw an unsurprisingly high number of white people die from 'tropical' disease (Arnold 1993; Patterson 1987).

By the late nineteenth century, the English affection for gin and tonic to ward off malaria and other tropical malaise also signified an increased knowledge of tropical medicine (Arnold 1996; Manderson 1996; Rosenthal 2001). Biomedicine, by this time an arm of the colonial project, was associated with enlightenment and modernity; traditional medicines and transcendental medicines were constructed as backward and unscientific. However, the rhetoric of biomedicine did not match its practice and far from colonizing the 'natives', was itself largely confined to the British military until the early twentieth century (Harrison 1994). Multiple factors – a bubonic plague in the 1890s, advances in medical science and sanitary practice, growing Indian involvement and the rise of the women's medical movement – forced biomedicine by the 1920s and 1930s to look beyond the barrack walls of the British army to the Indian population (Harrison 1994). This was helped along by the Indian Congresses' Nehruvian zeal for science and technology as a symbol of progress and development (Arnold 1996). These were the foundations of contemporary health technologies – such as diagnostics and testing (e.g., the MRI) and transnational health services (e.g., transcription services for doctor's notes) – and the means by which boundaries were defined between 'real' doctors (who were *au fait* with technology) and 'quacks'.

Transcendental medicine, which was seen as quackery and superstition, irrational and preying upon the ignorance of the masses, was delegitimized and cast out of institutionalized medicine by the early twentieth century, although it continues to echo in medical practice (Khan 2006; Khare 1996). Traditional medicine suffered a similar albeit less devastating fate. It was progressively 'unmade', increasingly seen as 'unscientific' through chronic underfunding of its training and research practices and was subject to intense regulation and bureaucratization. It was no coincidence that the de-professionalization of traditional medicine was concomitant with a growing preference among India's elite for biomedicine and this changed the traditional practitioner's clientele from the ruling to the poorer classes (Bala 2007; Leslie 1976).

Despite attempts at revival by Indian Nationalists (such as Gandhi), this trend continued. A small but significant scholarship describes how traditional medicine continued to be dismantled by the state after Independence (see Banerji 1981; Jeffery 1988; Khan 2006; Nandy 1995). It is only recently (from 1995 onwards) that traditional medicine has been institutionalized, with the establishment of the Department of *Āyurveda*, Yoga and Naturopathy, *Unani, Siddha* and Homoeopathy (AYUSH) within the Ministry of Health and Family Welfare (Government of India).

The Doctor-Patient Relationship: Past and Present

Don Bates (1995) suggests that the fundamental difference between Galenic medicine (biomedicine) and *Āyurveda* (traditional medicine) is the approach of the two to knowledge and knowing. Biomedicine privileges the 'epistemic' or the methods by which knowledge is created, constituted and certified, whereas traditional (and transcendental) medicine favours 'gnostic' knowing, which entails knowledge gained through initiation, experience and elaboration. Epistemic knowledge is about expertise. In contrast, gnostic knowledge is about the expert (Bates 1995). These pedagogical differences are critical to understanding how doctors in all three systems are perceived in India.

Historically, the doctor, known as the *vaid* in *Āyurveda* and as the *ḥakīm* in *Unani*, was perceived as a healer and holy man who combined theology and everyday living advice in his treatment. More than the patient, the onus was on the healer to lead a moral life. Vāgbhata in AD 600 wrote in his *Aṣṭāṅgahrdaya* or *The Heart of Medicine*, the preeminent text on Indian medicine: 'The physician is skilful, educated in the discipline by a master, has practical experience and is pure. . . . The patient is wealthy, obedient to the physician, informative and has endurance' (as translated by Wujastyk 2003: 209).

The purity, skill and pedigree of the healer created an expectation that the *vaid* was omniscient and wholly trustworthy and the patient, bolstered by wealth and fortitude, was to behave meekly and gratefully (von Schmädel and Hochkirchen 1987). This dominant-subordinate relationship was bound in class politics as most healers were Brahmans, a literate, priestly class who saw themselves as closer to God than most patients, who tended to be poorer and from a lower class (Trawick 1995). Ethics and consent, within this didactic relationship, were situational and implicit, i.e., by virtue of coming to the healer the patient and his family tacitly agreed to participate in the therapeutic encounter. The family was meant to place complete trust in the *vaid* and follow whatever he recommended. However, this was not a cessation of patient power, for the healer, as designated arbiter of morality and medicine, still had to forge an ethical therapeutic strategy that retained the patient's trust and gave him or her hope (Khare 1996). It was accepted that patients who felt ill-treated could go elsewhere and many did so, thus illustrating that doctor shopping has always been a part of the Indian therapeutic landscape.

In contrast, biomedicine sought to divorce the doctor-patient encounter from its context, exacerbating its dramaturgical nature and the autonomy of each actor. As traditional and transcendental medicine explicitly situated themselves within a mêlée of social and class relations (Finkler 1994) this created a disjuncture, one which was resolved by the 'Indianization' of biomedicine along the practitioner-patient praxis. Thus a 'good' doctor was (and is) one who personally engages with his patients (Gould 1965; Khare 1996).

Central to forging a meaningful engagement between doctor and patient was hope. Research done elsewhere shows that hope and the possibility of recovery is critical in formulating a relationship between doctor and patient, even when the possibility of recovery or return to normality is slight (Del Vecchio Good et al. 1994; Mattingly 1994; Warren and Manderson 2008).

A loose interpretation must be made of the word 'doctor' here, for based on my observations, people who were associated in an official capacity with a health service, irrespective of their qualification and experience, were cognisant of the responsibility and power invested in them. 'Say something positive', I was instructed by the local ARDSI volunteer when I visited Kottayam in rural Kerala. I had just met a poor woman, Gerriamma (75), conscious of her fading memory and desperate for a cure. Her unsuccessful dealings with allopathic, *Āyurvedic* and homeopathic medicines had been replaced by daily visits to the Church. She repeatedly asked me for a cure, whereupon I was given this instruction. Similarly, in Delhi, I observed a volunteer debating the healing successes of a popular Guru with the Mukherjee family. The volunteer discussed the Guru's daily television programme which showed miraculous cures for chronic ailments (no cases of failure were mentioned) and outlined his own fitness regime of a walk and yogic breathing exercises every morning.

Neither case was about peddling a commercial agenda nor about privileging particular medical systems. Rather, these reflected a tendency among people to give hope to families, which itself was emblematic of their frustration at the lack of an *ilāj* to cure this degenerative disease. Similar findings were made in Thailand (see Bennett 1999), where the truth about terminal illnesses was 'softened' by doctors, family members and the patients themselves. Dying was never discussed and even till the end stages, promises of a cure circulated. The underpinning rationale was to protect patients' psychological integrity and give them hope. Antonella Surbone reminds us, 'We all have a responsibility towards hope . . . and that it [hope] does not need to have "cure" as its object' (1997: 74 and 79).

The alternative of profound hopelessness is never really an option. When doctors failed to give hope or were challenged by their patients, reprimand was swift, as was illustrated in a Delhi *sarkari* (government hospital) OPD:

> A woman in her 60s has come to get her script refilled. She is well dressed in a clean pink and lavender sari, her grey hair is combed and coiled into a bun. Dr. Kumar eliminates some of her medication and she begins to protest, '*Sugar hai, heart ke leya hai*' [for my diabetes, for my heart]. Dr. Kumar replies that these medications are not related to her illnesses and one should not take medications *befikaar mei* [unnecessarily]. She continues to protest and the doctor gets irritated and yells at her: '*Tu khud apna ilāj kar le. Hamaree baat to tu maanne ko tayar nehi hai . . . jaao!*' [You cure yourself. You're not ready to accept our advice. Go!]. Kumar says this twice in the ensuing argument. He isn't going to fill her script or write or sign off on anything. Who was the doctor here – him or her? If she was so convinced that these medicines were essential, then why had she come to him? She should just treat herself. *Chhor* [forget it], he wasn't signing off on anything (*Field notes, 29th February 2008*).

Within these expectations and enforcement – of how patients should behave in an OPD, how volunteers should relate to families and how positive a researcher should be – lives India's medical history. Morality and power are vested in health authorities within pluralistic systems where clinicians, such as Dr Kumar, wield considerable power. In the above vignette we may read an example of 'medical dominance', a term that refers to the power that doctors exercise because of their clinical roles in diagnosis and treatment, ability to supervise the work of other health professionals and the privileged status of medicine compared to other health professions (Freidson 1970). A key feature of medical dominance is the autonomy that doctors enjoy. According to Freidson (1970: 135), 'His [doctor's] determinations are not subject to direct evaluation or review by another occupation: they may be limited by purely administrative or financial decisions made by others, but they may not be directly questioned except by other physicians'. But castigating the clinical approach of Dr Kumar, using the medical dominance paradigm, presupposes that he is in the business of domination not doctoring. In fact Kumar, as a doctor, represents medicine's capacity to offer an *ilāj* and hope to people. This is why doctors are held in such high esteem and patients want to consult them. Medicine's capacity to enhance human productivity also explains why it has been subsumed by the state, invested with power and appropriated at various points in history to control the masses (Foucault 1975). No doctor-patient relationship occurs in a clinical vacuum (Navarro 1976). Rather, in the politics of talk between Dr Kumar and his patient, existing social hierarchies are reinforced through the methods of communication (authoritarian subordinate) and the institutional settings (resource poor) in which this conversation occurs. The protocols around behaviour and authority are stringently adhered to with punitive consequences for those who baulk at these unwritten rules (Pinto 2004). As Navarro (1978, 1982, 1988) has argued, medicine reproduces the class, gender and race power relations of the wider society in which it operates. The task is to understand the wider political and economic forces that frame these clinical encounters.

'You Have to Be a Little Bit Mad to Work in a Place like This'

'The only thing that there is no shortage of around here is people', says Yashaswini drily. She sits behind her desk, tall and stern, neurologist first and woman second. She wears little makeup, minimal jewellery and comfortable shoes. Even her sari swishes in an orderly way beneath her white lab coat when she strides. She has a brusque, booming voice that she uses to demand for systematic administrative processes, for patients to come into her OPD room, for good quality drugs and treatment, for social workers to help poor families and for laboratory technicians to produce cleaner and better reports.

She sees approximately 1000 patients and their families per month from places such as Bihar (47 per cent literacy), Jharkhand (53.56 per cent literacy), Uttar Pradesh (56.27 per cent literacy) and Jammu and Kashmir (55.52 per cent literacy) (Census of India 2001, 2006). These are small town people fretting over their children's epilepsy (60 per cent of cases), their relative's head injuries (20 per cent), their own psychosomatic complaints (10 per cent) and their parents' dementia (less than 10 per cent). Yashaswini brusquely assesses them, 'Answer properly! When we ask you questions, if this is the sort of answers you give, then what will we do? We'll treat him accordingly. You people also!'

Patients, families, pharmaceutical representatives, hospital administrative staff and other doctors troop in and out of her OPD as she grows more irritable, '*Haa, haa* just barge in, we are all sitting in here having a party. Wait outside please, I will call you'. An attendant guards the door, a human blocker to humanity's clamour for an *ilāj*. Her OPD consultancy room is meagre: a desk, two chairs and a cold metal stool on which patients sit when they are examined. Three plastic chairs line one wall, an examination table covered by a dusty paint splattered blue sheet rests against the adjacent wall and nestled in the far corner is a basin with a shabby soap dispenser.

Yashaswini works hard and tries to improve the system. A family from Patiala has been waiting for six months to get the results of an MRI of their son's brain and she tells them to complain formally. A private MRI facility provides poor quality images at high prices so she telephones and yells at them, threatening to report them to the health authorities. When patient files go missing, as they often do, the File-in-Charge[5] opens new ones at her behest (OPD patient records are written not computerized). A family explains that the medication she prescribed was not available so the chemist gave them an alternative. She is infuriated: 'Do you know that nearly 50 per cent of the drugs available in the market are illegal? They don't do what they claim to. God knows what effect they have and they're not even registered. Who knows what *desi dava:i*[6] [local medicine] you've picked up and brought here? It doesn't even come in a box, they're selling it to you loose and you're giving it! I'm writing this again, you please buy it and don't substitute it with anything else'. She writes 'no substitute' on the script as well.

Yashaswini's story is neither unique nor particularly dysfunctional for a *sarkari* hospital. By comparison with other OPDs I visited, where between 150 and 200 patients would be seen in about two hours by four or five doctors, her OPD was organized and efficient. Usually only about 40 to 50 patients were seen in the course of two hours. The concerns she confronted – high patient demand, few resources, work overload, hospital bureaucracies, inferior quality tests and drugs – were themselves symptomatic of India's public health infrastructure (Jeffery 1988), which, like the public health systems of most developing nations, is shaped by the forces of class, history, globalization and institutional power.

Delhi has 131 *sarkari* hospitals[7] and 752 private facilities.[8] Yashaswini works at a premier teaching hospital, but in comparison to the private hospitals, hers is under-resourced and grappling with the health needs of millions of poor Indians who cannot afford private biomedical healthcare. Approximately 1.5 million outpatients and 80,000 inpatients are seen here every year. Concurrently, the number of *sarkari* doctors is dropping. The Planning Commission of India (2007) estimates a 600,000 shortfall in doctors across the country, a figure that is projected to increase as more registered doctors emigrate and students opt into higher paying jobs in engineering and business. Presently, an estimated 100,000 Indian doctors work in the US, the UK, Canada and Australia (Government of India 2006) – by some accounts, the largest émigré physician workforce in the world (Mullan 2006).

Patients in *sarkari* hospitals typically spend long hours waiting only to have less than two minutes with the doctor and interruptions during the consultation are common. This depressing finding has been reiterated since the 1970s (Das and Das 2006; Jeffery 1988; Murthy and Parker 1973;

Seth 1973) and is symptomatic of the skewed doctor-patient ratio nationwide (6.5:10,000) (WHO 2013). Additionally, the socially enforced behaviour for *sarkari* patients, wherein they have to be obsequious, cooperative and mild, has been linked to pressure for 'voluntary' gifts and informal payments for hospital admissions, bed availability and subsidized drugs (Jeffery 1988; Peters and Muraleedharan 2008). While I never observed such exchanges or such pressures in Yashaswini's OPD, patients were nevertheless dissatisfied with their experiences:

> In a government hospital it is not a happy situation, it is a depressing situation. Taking mummy there that day was really excruciating. It was the end of February and sitting there on those uncomfortable chairs from morning to evening, for me, I suppose it is ok but at her age, she is not used to it, it is terrible... I don't know how things are organized, the doctor comes, then suddenly they disappear and they come back. What they do – whether they have to take their rounds of the wards at that time – I don't know. The management and the discipline is hopeless, really, really hopeless (*Nayantara Sen, 58*).

Yet for doctors like Yashaswini, who choose to remain in *sarkari* hospitals, work is a gruelling twelve-hour day, seven days a week, with only every alternate Sunday off. Subsequently, her health, clinical and interpersonal skills are affected. She knows she cannot adhere to any imaginary gold standard:

> It is not like the West where you see two or three patients and you spend an hour and a half with each patient. You cannot do that. You don't have time to spend. It's probably the first evaluation which is the most detailed and after that it's more of a short amount of time that we can give them. The major challenge is time management for patients, time management for your own work, your own research, your family . . .

Yashaswini experienced migraines, conjunctivitis, dark rings under the eyes and lethargy during the months I sat in her OPD. When we finally had our interview in her clean air conditioned office, she was harried and hungry. Her answers were fired like bullets interspersed by people who stormed in and out, yelling about admissions, MRIs and bed availability. She yelled back. As I left, she smiled wryly and stated candidly, 'You have to be a little bit mad to work in a place like this'.

What Role for Human Rights?

For patients and their families who have to be admitted into a *sarkari* hospital, the experience is an ordeal. The hospital hierarchy positions patients at the bottom rung and privileges the institutional relationship between hospital and patient over the familial relationship between carers and people with dementia. When Harinder Singh (60) was admitted into the neurology ward by Yashaswini, only his wife Jaspreet was allowed into the ward with him. His son Ajit was told by the ward security guard, 'He is our patient and if you go up, you will disturb all the other patients'. Consequently Jaspreet was left to deal singlehandedly with her husband's wandering and incontinence.

> They just washed their hands of us . . . He wouldn't stay in bed and every 10 minutes he was doing his bathroom on the bed and this became a big concern. Sometimes he would get on someone else's bed, or touch someone else's bottle, [and] the whole day I was with him trying to manage this.

The ward staff gave Jaspreet two bed sheets and when Harinder soiled them, she was asked to wash them. When she requested a rubber sheet or a condom catheter, she was refused and told to take Harinder to the toilet. Meanwhile, Ajit would wait for hours in the hospital foyer, with food his sisters had prepared, periodically telephoning his increasingly hungry mother. The guard would not allow him to give the food to Jaspreet and when mother and son met at the entrance of the ward, the guard monitored them so closely that Jaspreet had to ask him to step back. Finally, after two days, Jaspreet had had enough:

> After all of this distress I said, 'We can take better care of him at home' and we brought him back. He made such a mess that for two to three days after I brought him back I was still washing his clothes. There how would I wash his clothes? They wouldn't let someone else stay with him, so how could I leave him and do it? I would just change him and put the soiled clothes in a plastic bag.

The family were angry and embittered by their experience. Harinder had picked up an infection while in the ward, which gave him severe diarrhoea and the family were still managing this when I went to visit them nearly two weeks after he had been discharged. Additionally, his balance had been affected following a spinal tap and he periodically fell down. But the Singh family's anger was directed at the guard.

The guard, a real and symbolic embodiment of institutional authority, is also an indicator of the depth of medical dominance in India, which is enacted at all levels of the biomedical institution. Yet, the Singh family's frustration with him reflects lay people's impatience with those who wield authority without knowledge. Ward guards, administrative staff, door attendants in OPDs and hospital clerks were perceived by families and patients as having the same social status as them, not in terms of class, caste or income, but in terms of knowledge – they knew nothing of the *ilāj* – and therefore their power was continuously undermined by patients who would argue and barge past them into the doctor's office. Doctors, nurses and occasionally doctoral researchers occupied a different power terrain because of the knowledge people believed they possess. As a result, I could squeeze into a crowded OPD while 200 people waited outside, or dismissively stride past a guard into the neurology ward on account of the status afforded to me. Class is always implicated in this dynamic, reflecting the power and capacity of some, more than others, to pursue doctoring, doctorates and other symbols of institutional power. Nita Kumar illustrates this well in an account of her dealings with the Varanasi police in the early 1990s: 'My clothes, coolness and confidence in going up to the doorman immediately marked me as someone from the top rather than from the bottom classes and everyone in such circumstances is judged by these things' (1992: 221).

The clothes and the lack of confidence of the Singhs marked them as unimportant to the guard and they were treated accordingly. Such judgements chalk out inequities and deny access to care for those who need it the most. Such blatant disrespect for the rights and dignity of people is symptomatic of what Paul Farmer (2003) has termed the 'pathologies of power', the structural violence that permits such human rights violations.

'We Fail Them'

Four pharmaceutical drugs are recommended for the treatment of dementia – donepezil (Aricept®), galantamine[9] (Reminyl®), rivastigmine (Exelon®) and memantine (Admenta®) (Alzheimer's Australia 2008). The first three drugs are cholinesterase inhibitors that aim either to increase levels of acetylcholine (an important neurotransmitter for memory) or strengthen nerve receptiveness to acetylcholine.

Among the twenty people with dementia who formed part of this study, there was an approximately equal use of donepezil, rivastigmine and memantine (see Figure 3.1). A prescription for medication was usually obtained following diagnosis, with follow-up visits every three to six months to *sarkari* OPDs for script refills. In theory, these visits were to monitor the disease progression, review and adjust the medication and counsel the family on what to expect next. The person experiencing dementia was meant to be seen by the doctor at least once a year. In practice however, people with dementia rarely returned to the OPD following diagnosis and

72 UNFORGOTTEN

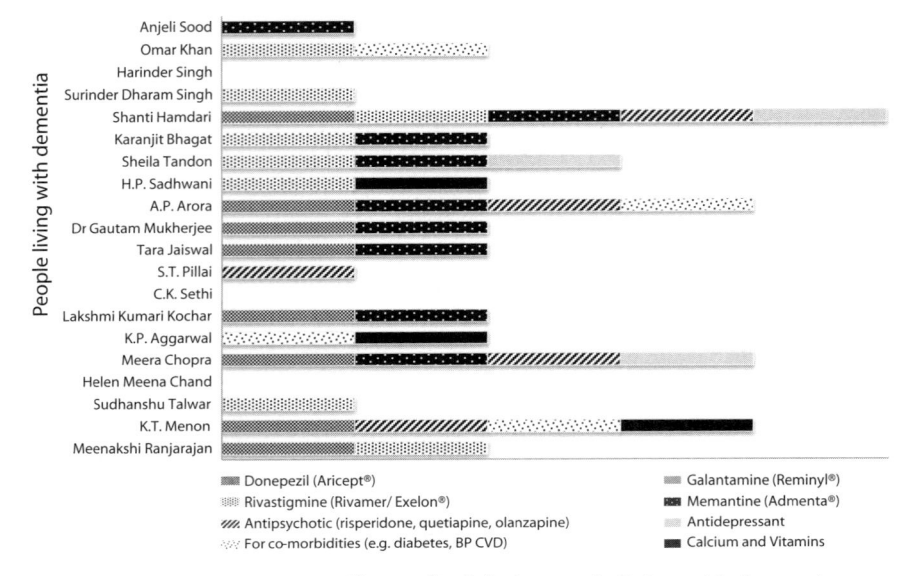

FIGURE 3.1 Concurrent use of biomedical *ilāj* by people living with dementia

instead their relatives would go to refill their scripts. Few got the opportunity to speak to the doctor, due to time restraints and competing patient demands.

Doctors generally signed the refill prescription while signing a host of other scripts without reviewing or adjusting the medication. Consequently, many people with dementia were on medications whose dosages had not been altered for years and/or were on antipsychotic medications that should have not been administered for more than a few months. Mrs Hamdari, for example, had been put on olanzapine (an antipsychotic drug approved for treatment of Bipolar I disorder and schizophrenia) following a bout of aggressive behaviour wherein she had slapped her maid. Although olanzapine was marketed off label for dementia patients (Spielmans 2009), in August 2008 it was shown to increase mortality among dementia patients by 1.6 to 1.7 times compared to those who were on a placebo (Lilly USA LLC 2009). When I first met Mrs Hamdari, in April 2008, it had been more than eighteen months since her first dosage. Her aggression had dissipated and she was experiencing increased levels of lethargy and drowsiness. Her daughter Nayantara attributed this change to the medication and was becoming increasingly concerned about the side effects but did not feel confident about adjusting the dosages on her own.

Finally in July 2008, with prompting from me, Nayantara returned to Yashaswini to ask for the medication to be reviewed, whereupon olanzapine was removed. Though I was able to intervene on behalf of Mrs Hamdari, most families navigate this field on their own. Among the sample, Mrs Hamdari was on the most medication, but the symptoms she experienced were part of an iatrogenic litany reported by families and key service providers. Again and again, families complained of the nausea, diarrhoea, aggression, weeping, drooling and unsteady gait that the person with dementia experienced as a result of taking cholinergic inhibitors drugs and antipsychotic medications.

Few families reported any positive effects; only K.L. Chopra felt his wife Meera had improved, i.e., was calmer, with medication. Many, like Nandini Pillai, felt that antipsychotic drugs made caring more difficult:

> His [father] life changed completely in the sense that even his gait wasn't steady and he was drooling and obviously what he was saying wasn't very clear. There were times that he fell, the number of times that he fell ... There was a time I went to the market, came back and he was sitting under the tap waiting for me to come home to lift him up. Once he locked himself inside the bathroom and we had to call the carpenter to break open the door.

Typically the deleterious effects of medications far outweighed any supposed benefit, not only physiologically, but also relationally. While the dementia undeniably and irretrievably changed relationships, the administration of medications tended to sharpen the carer's gaze on the body of the person living with dementia. When medications were administered (before or after meals), how it was administered (swallowed whole, crushed and disguised with food, chewed as it was) and the effects it had, such as increased nausea, sleepiness, drooling, all required carer input, surveillance and management of the body. Medicines became an embodiment of discipline for both carers and people with dementia. Giving and taking medicines were part of the routine of care, alongside activities such as feeding, bathing and exercising. ARDSI volunteer Somya Ghosh explained the disciplinary function of antipsychotic medications:

> Unfortunately I feel that there are some families who are very happy for the doctors to give antipsychotic drugs and make the person very numb and drowsy. That way the problems of wandering, the problems of lying, the problems of repeating oneself are gone. 'I can manage him this way. I am alone; I have to manage him this way. You tell me, what is my predicament? If I go to the doctor and stop all his medication and the person does all these things, then what do I do?' We sometimes don't know what answers to give, we fail them.

Yet, most carers baulked at privileging a docile physical body, achieved through medication, at the expense of social relations. Ultimately many reduced, or even stopped, the medication altogether. Curiously, this course of action was gendered: female carers tended to be ambivalent while male carers were zealous about medications. For women, medications were part of the caring gamut and this finding accords with work done on HIV/AIDS that found that for women living with HIV, drug regimens had an intrusive effect on everyday life and that social relations strongly influenced their ability to comply with medications (Johnston and Mann 2000; McDonald, Bartos and Rosenthal 2001).

Older women's experiences with medication administration are often problematized as 'adherence' and 'error' (Arlt et al. 2008; Col, Fanale and Kronholm, 1990; Sorensen et al. 2005). Such language obfuscates the complex decision making behind such 'errors' and fails to acknowledge the effect of adverse drug reactions. In the US, more people are admitted to hospitals for adverse drug reactions than non-compliance (Heath 2003), and in the UK about 11 per cent of hospitalized patients suffer an adverse drug reaction with greater risk of mortality following such an episode (Eaton 2002). In India, although pharmacovigilance has had a twenty-year history on paper, chronic underfunding has left it largely ineffectual in practice (Biswas and Biswas 2007). Nevertheless, Indian studies have shown that adverse drug reactions can and do happen, often with fatal consequences, and that older people are especially vulnerable (Malhotra et al. 2001; Ramesh, Pandit and Parthasarathi 2003).

In my study sample, only three people were not on any medication – Helen Meena Chand (who refused to take any) and C.K. Sethi and Harinder Singh (whose families opted not to give them any). However, only six women administered medications as a matter of course, while the rest sought alternatives elsewhere (n=6) or reduced the dosages of their own volition (n=5). None put great stock in the capacity of a biomedical *ilāj* and in some cases (n=5) doctors themselves discouraged these women from administering medicines. Vandhana Arora was candid about her expectations for her father-in-law:

> Basically we cannot expect any recovery from this. It [medicines] provides certain stability to the behaviour and maybe the progression is not very fast. But to expect recovery in a case like this is foolishness. I think more than the medicines, it is the handling of the patient which will direct his further behaviour and symptoms. It is a degeneration.

Men, in contrast, often tried to administer various medications to their wives. For them the pursuit of an *ilāj* – obtaining a script, getting a refill, buying the medication and offering and administering a range of pills – was a way of retaining control and performing *sevā*. Mr Chopra medicated his wife for all manner of ailments, much to the consternation of his sons and daughters-in-law. Shivbaksh Chand, the most recalcitrant and beguiling person I met in Delhi, had filled half of a small carton with an assortment of drugs, most in strips, with the packaging long lost. In his first interview, he declared that he and his wife Helen had dementia, 'but she more than me'. Whether this dementia was the irascibility of ageing, or a neuropathology that affected them both, or a hybridized dementia whereby he mimicked her symptoms to obtain treatment because she refused to leave her home, eluded me. I never managed to ascertain who had dementia and at what stage. Shivbaksh and Helen proved far too wily.

> I am eating my medicines. Look how many medicines I am taking every day. [High pitched voice] *So many medicines!*
> Yes that's why I am still alive [Riffles through box]. I am a blood pressure patient also; see these are the medicines I take for that. And see this medicine and this one . . . [Addresses his wife] What time of the day is it?
> Helen: it's daytime, around noon.
> [To BB] she's said the right thing. It's about to be 12 'o clock. [To Helen] Here eat this calcium tablet.
> Helen: No, I don't want it.

Shivbaksh took half his medicines and unsuccessfully attempted to feed Helen the rest. He was diagnosed in a *sarkari* OPD amid hundreds of other patients and had never visited a neurologist's office. He spent his days in search of many kinds of *ilāj* and once asked me to get his script refilled. When I returned with the refill, I discovered that I was not the only person that had been pressed into this service, for a young man from the main *Āyurvedic* dispensary in the adjacent suburb had also come to drop off medication. For Shivbaksh, medicines were a means of illustrating how much *sevā* he performed for Helen, even though she spurned all of the medications he brought her.

For Helen, medicines would prolong a life she had long grown weary of and she told me on two separate occasions of her desire to die. Thus, *ilāj* was both a cure and an imprisonment in this household, functioning as a disciplinary signifier by virtue of its social and chemical compositions. Chemically *ilāj* as a pharmaceutical drug could 'cure' or minimize the behavioural and psychological symptoms of dementia and so restore (to a degree) the normal social order of things, although in practice this was not the case. But these 'normal' social orders were also the disciplinary structures of Helen's life, which she resisted by doing no housework, refusing to leave her home, not seeing a doctor and not taking any medication. Pound and colleagues (2005) have argued that despite widespread belief in the benefit of drugs, individuals also resist consuming medicines in various ways (e.g., self-modification of dosages, symptomatic use only) because of the coercive power of drug regimens. Helen's resistance to all forms of *ilāj* was also a resistance to her life. She refused to be housewife and patient and sought to step outside the disciplinary project through death.

Avoiding death and degeneration was also the purpose of Govind Ballabh Tandon's life. Like Shivbaksh, he spent his days stoically searching for an *ilāj* for his wife Sheila, who was in the late stages of dementia. But in his final interview he tragically conceded:

> I consulted the doctor and all the doctors are of the opinion that the medicine works in the initial stage but is ineffective in the later stages. So whether you give it or not, it is useless. So for the past four months I have been reducing it. For five years I was increasing it and now I am reducing it . . . Within six months I want to stop all her medicines.

Reducing and ultimately stopping medications was for families an acceptance of the inevitability of death. This realization occurred with time as hope gradually faded. Hope is a central feature of the administration of any medication and for families, the hope for an *ilāj* was a driving force in their doctor shopping. This finding has a broader resonance with studies from the US (Lindstrom et al. 2006) and Canada (Rockwood, Graham and Fay 2002), which show that patients and families living with dementia hoped for improvements or at least stasis in function, cognition, leisure, behaviour and social interaction through medication. But when biomedical forms of *ilāj* failed to deliver, unlike in the Western context where doctors are meant to fight to the end, in India, both doctors and families were fully and freely able to recognize the role of God, religion and faith in the welfare of the person with dementia (Khare 1996). As the stories of Vandhana, Shivbaksh and Tandon illustrate, the search for *ilāj* is a combination of hope and desperation in the face of degeneration and chaos. Biomedicine is but one part of this broader search and traditional and transcendental medicines also play an important role in managing dementia.

Traditional Medicine and Temperance

Fourteen families used traditional medicines. Treatments from multiple traditional systems were often used simultaneously. *Āyurveda* and homeopathy were the most popular combination (n=10 and 8 respectively), but an assortment of other therapies such as yoga, acupuncture, reiki, herbal medicines and magnetic therapy were also used by families. Unlike in the West, where such therapies are accessed as 'alternatives' or 'complementary' to biomedicine (Astin et al. 1998), in India these treatments, reflecting a medically pluralist society, are accessed in conjunction and are administered alongside biomedicines (Tandon, Prabhakar and Pandhi 2002).

In India, in 2012, there were 720,937 registered traditional medical practitioners and 852,195 registered allopathic doctors (Department of AYUSH 2012; Medical Council of India 2012). Traditional practitioners are usually private practitioners and shoulder much of the burden of healthcare in rural India. Despite having a large presence in the Indian therapeutic landscape, there is a hierarchy of knowledge, with biomedicine ranked at the top. Traditional medicine is not viewed as analogous to biomedicine and so biomedical doctors accepted that their patients used traditional medicines and rarely discouraged them from doing so. But Yashaswini said:

> We don't discourage them from taking *Āyurvedic* or homeopathic, we just tell them that it should not have harmful metals. They do experiment. Some of them claim that they are better with these medicines.
> *What do you think?*
> I am sure that there is something there which works. It is only that we haven't investigated them in a scientific manner; these herbs are well known from ancient times. They could improve the memory. In fact research on turmeric, cumin and some of the herbs is going on in Western settings.

Ashis Nandy (1995) has argued that the appropriation of techniques and ingredients from traditional medicine by biomedicine is part of a process of delegitimizing these epistemologies by rendering them 'unscientific', while simultaneously absorbing, assimilating or marginalizing certain aspects of traditional medicine. Families have accepted this knowledge hierarchy and adjusted their expectations accordingly: traditional medicines were viewed as more suited to chronic disease management than biomedicine because, even though they were perceived as less effective, they had fewer side effects (see also Chacko 2003; Dalal 2000). For emergencies, biomedicine was still the first port of call, even among carers who were strong advocates for traditional medicines:

> If there is a crisis, like if there is a terrible chest infection, you have to give the antibiotics, there is no other way about it . . . Then it is best to take the person off the *Āyurvedic* medicine for that period because the antibiotic will do its work. So just take it off until the crisis is over and then get back on it for the chronic (*Namita Sood*, 53).

Intriguingly, traditional medicine's second-tier ranking bolstered its veracity in my study, as families had reduced expectations of an *ilāj* and therefore their dealings tended to be more fruitful. Namita Sood, Nandini Pillai, Nayantara Sen, Bhageshwari Srivastava and Nina Bhagat all put great stock in their homeopaths, herbalists and *Āyurvedic* doctors because none had promised an *ilāj* but all had managed to affect positive changes such as increased calm, improved functionality and greater energy among people with dementia. Nina said of Karamjit's treatment:

> Everything had gone *gheech-peech* [topsy-turvy], but this medicine we are giving him has brought his strength back. This herbal medicine, we are giving him a very powerful dose, which the astronauts take, so that he builds his inner strength up. Once he builds his inner strength he will have more confidence and if he starts playing good golf then he will ask his friends to play.

Two key points stand out in Nina's words: (1) the establishment of the potency and integrity of the herbal medicines by highlighting its use by astronauts; and (2) the effect of these medicines in improving relations, i.e., one can play good golf with friends. Both points are underwritten by class. All these carers were highly educated, English-speaking women, who resided in the wealthy suburbs of south Delhi. They were astute and gauged the effectiveness of their traditional doctors by the latter's professional qualifications and refusal to give hope. This contrasted with their experiences with biomedicine, from which they initially wanted hope and an *ilāj*. Those traditional practitioners who promised a cure were viewed with scepticism, as 'quacks' who made extraordinary claims. As a result families were dismissive:

> I've never met a homeopathic doctor who's said, 'We don't have the treatment for this disease'. Of all the doctors I've seen, the allopath ones will tell you, 'These are the medicines I have and whatever effect they have we'll see because there is no cure for this illness'. But the homeopaths, the number that we have seen, even the famous ones will say, 'With our medicines he'll be fine. Any day now he'll start playing football' (*Mamta Aggarwal, 38*).

If the power of biomedicine was undermined by the prudence of its doctors, then the power of traditional medicine rested on the circumspection of its practitioners. Such an equation reflects the location and professionalization of traditional medicine. By a refusal to give an *ilāj* traditional medicine distances itself from quackery and its claims to cure all. By Nina's comparison of the medicines with those that the astronauts take, one can see how traditional medicine seeks to yoke itself to scientific institutions and accrue legitimacy.

The professionalization of traditional medicines, most especially Āyurveda, commenced at the turn of the twentieth century when its practitioners sought to mimic biomedicine by establishing their own colleges, associations and pharmaceutical firms (Sivaramakrishnan 2006). If imitation is the best form of flattery, then such a move reaffirmed biomedicine's hegemony. But as Jean Langford (1999) points out, if professional Āyurveda is only partially reproductive of biomedicine, parody and challenge is also possible. Whether consciously or not, traditional medicine occupies both locales; it has borrowed heavily from biomedical diagnostic techniques through use of blood tests, histopathology, x-rays and stethoscopes, only then to prescribe its own treatment and disease etiologies. It also crosses into the domain of transcendental medicine in the way in which it mythologizes the savant-like capacity of some of its practitioners (Langford 1999, 2003). Shivanni, a homeopath, said:

> Here there are many quacks . . . That is why the reputation of homeopathy is a little down. Otherwise [there are] many well-known renowned homeopaths, [and if] you read their prescriptions, they are excellent. Even today there are some homeopaths who, when the patient enters the room, the medicine will come into their minds immediately. They have no need to ask them anything. If the patient speaks on his own they'll listen, but they've determined the medicine the moment the patient entered the room.

Traditional medicine's overlap with biomedicine and transcendental medicine has caused quiet rancour among some within the Ministry of Health and Family Welfare. Arvind Jaitley, a young but embittered bureaucrat, dismissed Āyurvedic and homeopathic medicine, questioning the efficacy of traditional medicine (or lack thereof as he saw it) and the methods used in diagnosis. 'Without a side effect is there any effect?' he argues. Jaitley worked in the mental health field and has a clinical qualification. A number of Āyurvedic medicine students had approached him to train them in psychiatric diagnostic techniques because there was no equivalent in Āyurveda. 'How can this [Āyurveda] be an effective science?' he said disbelievingly, 'yet there is a government ministry dedicated to it!' However, Jaitley's circumspection excluded critical reflection on contemporary diagnostics in mental health and the conditions under which diagnosis is made.

Unlike Jaitley, the Indian government and the WHO have increasingly recognized the potential of traditional medicine and have sought to incorporate traditional medicines into national health programmes and policy and to ensure the safety and efficacy of traditional medicines, their rational use and affordable access. Most families in my study were impressed by traditional medicine because of its effect in reducing the symptoms of social distress, such as aggression, wandering and listlessness. Where biomedical drugs created docile physical bodies at the expense of social relations, traditional medicines tempered the effects of biomedicine and facilitated the reintroduction of social relations. Nina said, 'Herbal medicine I will not recommend anyone, unless he or she is dedicated and the activities are followed – then it has effect'. Activities for Nina included reading, writing, counting, yoga, golf, massage, morning walks and hot and cold compresses for her husband Karamjit. Through all of these activities she could interact with him, monitor his development and adjust her strategies in her fight against his dementia.

Nina's story was one of some success and most families had positive experiences with traditional medicine. However, one man came away bitterly disappointed. Tandon had taken Sheila for 'acupuncture' treatments for nearly a year, only to find that she was deteriorating faster than he expected. He said:

> This man had promised me, 100 per cent to treat her. Whenever I go to a doctor the first thing I ask is whether it is possible to cure her or not. He had told me, 'Yes there is a cure and in 90 sittings she will be cured'. He was asking for Rs 1 lakh. I said, 'I'll give you a lakh but you give me a promise that she will be cured'.

This purported cure involved the insertion of about seventy needles into Sheila's head and neck, through which twenty volts of electricity would be passed for around thirty to forty-five minutes. Each sitting was about six hours and was very painful for her. During our first interview, Tandon showed me a video on his mobile phone of Sheila receiving the treatment. She repeatedly murmured, 'Go away, go away'. For Tandon, the failure of acupuncture was the failure of yet another *ilāj* – he had already tried biomedicine, *Āyurveda*, homeopathy and reiki. He had quit his job and reversed gender roles, spending his days searching for a cure, to no avail. He sought relief from his failure through self-analysis, watching TV, listening to music and playing games on the computer. Yet he never ceased hoping and, though a firm believer in science, he turned to religious healers for an *ilāj*.

Cosmopolitan Transcendental Medicine

At the core of religion and medicine is suffering, distress and disorder, a cry for help and salvation (Kleinman and Seeman 1999). Despite staking its claim in a rationalist discourse, medicine cannot escape its moral and soteriological dimensions. Suffering and salvation go to the heart of medicine, are woven throughout its history and praxis and manifest themselves in complex ways in daily life (Good 1994). If religion and medicine are so closely connected, then transcendental medicine, also known as 'religious healing', with its overt claims to religion and medicine, is an ambiguous hinterland. To try and separate religion and healing or medicine and the transcendent could well be like trying to separate the *dal* and rice from a *khichri*:[10] the two are inextricable. Nevertheless, I make this crude attempt, if only to distinguish between what families derived from the transcendent and transcendental medicine. The former was constructed by families as a prism through which meanings could be made while the latter was the source of a cure. Nearly all the families mentioned the role of God and religion in helping them build resilience, patience and strength in managing their loved one. Faith and resilience were the primary goals that families sought from religion. But transcendental medicine, while borrowing heavily from the mythologies of religion and culture, was where an *ilāj* was explicitly asked for. Here the purpose of the divine was not to relieve but to actively intercede through the medium of the religious healer. Such healers were thus presumed to be omniscient and able to deliver miracles.

The Khan family consulted a number of *jhāṛ-poṅch* practitioners (*jhāṛna* means to sweep or dust; *poṅchna* to wipe) in a bid to cure Omar's dementia. These practitioners are conventional sorcerers who conceive of illnesses as a result of curses or jealousies and seek to sweep or dust away these evils, often using brooms in their rituals. Illness as the effect of *kala jādū* (black magic) has a long history in folk medicines across the world, but what distinguishes the *jhāṛ-poṅch*, who the Khans consulted from other shamans and folk healers, was his recommendation that they also sacrifice a goat. This notion of sacrifice comes from the Qur'an, when Allah commanded Abraham to sacrifice that which he loved the most – his son – which Allah then replaced with a goat. The slaughter of the goat itself is symbolic, i.e., one sacrifices that to which one is closest and most attached; the fable itself is also significant in Judaic and Christian texts. Thus the Khan's *jhāṛ-poṅch* practitioner, along with his broom, combines mythology and literature in his treatment. Islamic transcendental medicine is of course far more complex than just these practices (see Cammann 1969; Gardner 1993; Pfleiderer 1988).

Only three families other than the Khans sought transcendental medicine: Nayantara, the Talwar family and Tandon. The Talwars had a prior relationship with their guru in south India, while the remaining healers were sought through personal referral. This is in line with Veena and Ranendra Das (2006), who point out that individual illness experiences are brokered through various filters and are contingent on what influence and treatment can be activated, rather than directed by a defined explanatory model for treatment (Kleinman 1980). Three families came to transcendental medicine in an ad hoc manner – extended family entreated Shafia Khan to visit the *jhāṛ-poṅch* practitioner, a friend mentioned Dr Francis to Nayantara and Tandon came across Guru Ramdev through the media.

Nayantara and the Talwars felt they had had some success, not so much in the outcomes for the people with dementia, but more from the sense of peace they derived from visiting their healers. While this skirts along the borders of the priest-parishioner relationship, the families' curative goals and the nature of the interactions were distinct from those of religious pastoral care. There was the notion of a magical 'healing touch' – the Talwars, for example, believed that after their guru raised his right palm towards seventy-eight-year-old Sudhanshu, his dementia halted and there had been no deterioration since. Similarly Nayantara said of her faith healer Dr Francis:

> When you're near to him, [it's] very calm and peaceful and it's very nice. You barely stand for a fraction of a moment, he just does this [raises her palm and moves it in a circle]. He makes you sit down if you have a photograph and he said that mummy's phosphorous level is very low. He is a doctor, in the sense that he is an allopath but he has studied many, many alternative medicines, he's been all over the world.

Just as traditional medicine challenges biomedicine through imitation and divergence, transcendental medicine challenges biomedicine and traditional medicine. Nayantara's experiences with Dr Francis highlight again the relationship between credibility, medicine and healing. Dr Francis' credibility rests in his status as an allopathic doctor and in his knowledge of alternative medicines. He is both spiritual healer and world traveller, combining the historicity of the doctor-patient relationship in India and a claim to authenticity that rests on globalization.

The established autocratic healer-patient relationship, which predated the arrival of biomedicine in India, was reflected in Nayantara's perception of Dr Francis. Like the *vaids* of old, the purity of Dr Francis' character and the peaceful feelings he engendered became the foundation of his healing powers (his magical touch) and these in turn influenced the time he gave to Nayantara, 'a fraction of a moment', and her acceptance of this very limited interaction. Broader issues of class and globalization were also implicit in this dynamic, not only in the resources that Dr Francis mobilized to travel around the world and educate himself, but also in the location of his practice in an exclusive south Delhi market. This market, favoured by the European expatriate population, is surrounded by elite suburbs in which diplomats, politicians and wealthy industrialists lived.

While Dr Francis did not directly charge his clients (it was up to them to make a donation on every visit), given his location he must have made a tidy profit.

Yet, in comparison with other religious healers, Dr Francis' ambit was minuscule. There are much larger enterprises at work, as Tandon discovered when he went to the holy city of Haridwar, a therapeutic beacon in north India, layered with religion, morality, healing and money. Tandon's excursion to Haridwar was to see Guru Ramdev, founder of the Divya Yog Mandir Trust which promotes yoga and *Āyurvedic* treatments. Ramdev is rich and famous. He created a transcendental medicine corporation which sells its own pharmacopeia of drugs based on his recipes and an assortment of DVDs on yoga. He has TV shows on yoga that are screened in India and abroad and holds yoga camps worldwide, including one at the residence of the President of India (Yoga Headlines India 2009). Ramdev's global popularity reflects the multiple beliefs that people from the subcontinent have in relation to experiences of health and illness, the range of practitioners they seek as a consequence and the falseness of the assumption that only people with low levels of education access such practitioners – findings that other studies have also made (Rao 2006; Rhodes et al. 2008; Small et al. 2005).

Ramdev's followers claim to have been cured from cancer, hepatitis and obesity, among other diseases. Tandon's reasons for visiting him were grounded in this political economy and the ready availability of his medicines:

> I didn't meet him. He doesn't meet you, his *hakīm* meets you. His prescribed his medicines and they are available in Delhi also. I took her for a consultation so that afterwards whatever medicines Ramdev has given, I can buy.

Alongside the consumption and marketing of *ilāj* and doctor-patient relations that frame it, medical pluralism in India is again illustrated. Guru Ramdev, whose practices and treatments derive from Hindu philosophy and who is located in a holy Hindu city, has a *hakīm* (*Unani* doctor, Islamic origins) and not a *vaid* (*Āyurvedic* doctor, Hindu origins) to dispense medicines. Even if Tandon had conflated the terms, the intermingling of different religions by practitioners and patients is evident. Transcendental medicine in India is not contained as specific denominations do not go only to their particular religious healer, i.e., Hindus to *vaids*, Muslims to *hakīms*, nor have national borders ever stopped this flow (Alter 2005). Rather these are polysynthetic systems where people access a variety of healers based on their perceived credibility and power. So Nayantara, a Hindu Brahmin, went to Dr Francis, a Christian; Tandon went to Guru

Ramdev who employed *hakīms* and not *vaids*; and the Khans consulted a *jhāṛ-ponch* practitioner who told them to sacrifice a goat based on a tale that has Islamic, Christian and Judaic roots.

Conclusion

Ilāj in its etymological, physiological and relational definitions has been used to contextualize the history of medical pluralism and the current state of play in India. Shaped by trade and colonization, class politics and scholastic and geographic epistemologies, medicine in India is segmented into biomedicine, traditional and transcendental medicine, which play out in urban and rural environs, public and private settings, in different and multiple ways. When searching for an *ilāj* for dementia, families operate within this landscape through doctor shopping and through concurrent engagement with different systems. These engagements are both exploitative and edifying: the *sarkari* doctor's indifference due to patient demands and few resources, the traditional doctor's greed and ignorance and the faith healer's arrogance and futility are balanced against the positive effects they generate, whether it is in Yashaswini constantly striving to improve her hospital, the increased interactions that Nina enjoys with Karamjit, or the sense of peace that Nayantara derives from visiting Dr Francis.

I have tried to show that through all of these transactions, the search for an *ilāj* is also a search for a 'good' doctor. Cure and social relations go hand in hand in India and, unlike in the West, most health practitioners here are cognisant and tolerant of this search. The doctor-patient relationship, which has historically been regimented and dictatorial, is increasingly challenged by families, people living with dementia, academics and the state. There is a long way to go in achieving a more equitable alignment of relations and this itself is bound within larger power plays of money and agency. The direct costs associated with the pursuit of an *ilāj* have not been explored and will be untangled in the following chapter. It is sufficient at this point to note that these costs are objective and subjective and that families have to dig deep monetarily and emotionally to pay them.

To date there is no cure for Alzheimer's disease or any age related dementia. Degeneration and death are inevitable. For many this is hard to accept and some never entirely give up hoping for a cure. For people like Tandon, finding a cure is the defining purpose of his days. He had two large plastic bags filled with papers containing information on Sheila's medical history, his correspondence with doctors all over the world, journal articles on cholinesterase inhibitors, newspaper cuttings and so on. His investigations were an emotional quest and he continuously reiterated his need to 'remain hopeful, to be positive, to have positive thinking'. He believes that a cure will be found, that the disease can be reversed, that dead cells can somehow be recharged. But he is anxious about whether the cure will be found in time for Sheila. In the deep corners of his heart and mind, he knows this probably will not happen. In my last interview with him, as I was walking out of the door, I stopped:

Cough. Beware of cough. If that happens it could progress into something more.
I know. It [cough] could mean a respiratory infection, a chest infection and that comes at the last stage. That will happen in the end.
I know you don't think doctors are very cooperative but you need to think about what you want to do then. A hospital's job is to keep the patient alive at all costs. One of my people ended up in the hospital and there were feeding tubes and oxygen and everything else. The other died in his bed at home. Whatever you think about either, you need to think about what outcome you want for her.
[Nods and smiles] I know this, I am aware. But I have to be positive, I have to have hope. Positive thinking is what I must do.

Notes

1. Although I only cite *Āyurveda* and *Unani* in this section, traditional medicine is much broader and, according to the Indian Ministry of Health and Family Welfare, includes *Āyurveda*, Yoga and Naturopathy, *Unani*, *Siddha* and Homoeopathy.
2. The Dharmashastra texts are a set of treatises developed between 200 BC and AD 200 that lay out the fundamental principles of living and modes of behaviour or dharma for every living creature, every kind of human being and each stage of life through which a man transits to and from (Trawick 1995). According to the *Manusmriti*, the most famous of these texts, there are four classes of men: the *brahmanas* (brahmins) (serving as priests and teachers), *kshatriyas* (duties of administration, battle and law enforcement), *vaishyas* (customarily agriculture, commerce and cow protection) and *shudras* (who provide service to members of the other three classes) (Kane 1930, 1962; The Laws of Manu c. 500 BC).
3. A *guru* is a teacher, mentor and spiritual guide. A *baba* was the head of the order of monks called Calendars or *Qalandar*, but the term is used nowadays to refer to all manner of *fakirs*. *Pīrs* refers to Muslim saints.
4. A *tabeez* is an amulet with an inscription from the Qur'an meant to ward off curses and djinns.
5. English term for an administrative clerk who manages patient records and files; the term is spoken in English even if the remainder of the sentence is in Hindi.
6. *Desi dava:i* is used to refer to the range of indigenous medicines which may be included in traditional medicine. Colloquially, it is also used with reference to the

efficacy of such medicines and the ad hoc manner in which they are manufactured and distributed. *Desi dava* may also be unregistered, unlisted medicines, which may be sold by pharmacists, traditional practitioners and religious healers.
7. See http://www.delhi.gov.in/wps/wcm/connect/d4c513804c2c319f81b0859 991226613/53+-+64+Medical.pdf?MOD=AJPERES&lmod=-617270539&CAC HEID=d4c513804c2c319f81b08599991226613 (accessed on 16 December 2013).
8. This figure is based on the number of private facilities recognized by the Government of the National Capital Territory of Delhi; the actual number of private hospitals may be higher.
9. At the time of interviewing, galantamine was not legally marketed in India.
10. *Khichri* is made by boiling lentils and rice together. It closest equivalent is a risotto in Italian cooking. To clarify the analogy, trying to separate religion and religious healing is like trying to separate the egg and oil in mayonnaise.

4. THE ECONOMIES OF CARE

I USE THREE CONCEPTS TO analyse the economy of dementia care in India – cost, identity and exchange. Cost is understood as the value associated with the material objects used in care (e.g., medicines, diapers, catheters) and the subjectivities of care (e.g., physical and emotional health of carers). Subjective costs, I argue, are hidden costs, tied to the marketplace and emotional work of care. These are the costs to the personhood of carers and the people with dementia: those secret tallies that either render identity ambiguous and uncertain, or reinforce existing notions of identity.

Commoditizing care, whether within the home or in the public sphere, involves exchanges that are commercial, reciprocal and redistributive (Polanyi 1957). I explore the exploitative relationships between institutions, carers and paid attendants but also the hidden benefits of the institutional costs of care, the pharma-economy of care and the domestic politics within households where paid attendants are employed to care.

Ultimately what will become visible is that even when carers engage in practices of consumption that are assumed to be beneficial to them, there are always costs to be paid by someone. In documenting the economies of care and its effects, this chapter is intentionally negatively oriented. This is not to deny the positive side of carework, which I address later. Rather, I emphasize the various tolls of care as I firmly believe if a complete picture is to emerge of dementia care in urban India today, then our analysis must include the shadows as well as the light.

'This is Not a Disease for the Poor'

In 2010, based on a global prevalence of 35 million people with dementia, the estimated costs of care were US$604 billion. The cost of informal care was US$251.8 billion, direct medical care was US$96.4 billion and the direct social costs were US$255.6 billion. Although 70 per cent of these total costs were incurred in Europe and North America, even in developing nations such as India the costs were huge. The most recent figures from South Asia, based on a prevalence of 4.4 million people with dementia in 2010, estimated the total costs (direct medical costs + costs of informal care + direct social costs) at approximately US$4 billion (Wimo et al. 2013). As India's prevalence rate is expected to grow by more than 300 per cent by 2040, there is a need for greater health investment and bolstering of health and care resources (Prince, Livingston and Katona 2007).

In the Eleventh Five Year Plan (2007–2012), the Government of India allocated Rs 128 crore (A$2.31 million)[1] to meet the health needs of its older citizens. The funds were earmarked for: (1) comprehensive preventative, curative and rehabilitation services for older people; (2) professional training and research in geriatrics and gerontology; and (3) the establishment of a National Institute for Ageing to coordinate health and ageing initiatives with other national health programmes (e.g., the Rural Health Mission) (Government of India 2007). The Twelfth Five Year Plan (2012–2017) revealed that Rs 74.2 crore had been spent and that the government's plans moving forward included: (1) setting up a National Commission for Senior Citizens, Bureau for Socio-Economic Empowerment of Senior Citizens and a National Trust for the Aged to ensure that health, social and economic services and facilities were being provided at national, state and district levels; (2) establishment of old age homes for indigent older people; (3) setting up help lines for older people; (4) provision of 'smart' identity cards for older people; and (5) provision of health insurance for older people (Government of India 2012).

But enmeshed within the legendary red tape of India's bureaucracy, these funds and initiatives will take time to reach communities. In 2007, three chapters of ARDSI – in Delhi, Kolkata and Chennai – secured government funds to set up day-care centres for people with dementia (ten to fifteen people per centre). When I arrived in January 2008, there were plans to locate an appropriate property for the new day-care centre in Delhi. When I left in October 2008, the location had been identified, but the funds had not yet been remitted and were still being filtered through central and state government departments. Midway through 2009, money and endeavour met and since then, the day-care centre in Delhi and more recently, a long-term dementia care facility in Faridabad has been in operation. Meanwhile other chapters have managed to establish their own day-care centres with funds sourced elsewhere. For some ARDSI workers, such as Somya Ghosh, advocating to the government was not worth the effort:

It's not in terms of fixing an appointment and talking, it's after that, how it gets taken care of. The file gets lost somewhere. Very frankly, we as an organization rely on local fundraising. We want local people to contribute to their community. Government funds are appreciated but we don't depend on them. You see, an organization like us, that is run by three to four people, to pursue a high government level – I don't know how many hours a job like that would be. We don't have time and if I have to spend an hour sitting at a window to get a pink pass to see a bureaucrat, I would not really be inclined to do that. In that time I would rather see a family.

Delays in transfer of government funds meant that these chapters were perennially underfunded, under-resourced and facing extinction – an ongoing concern for the vast majority of NGOs. ARDSI-DC's reliance on funding from government sectors and private donor agencies meant that their programs were often shaped by funding agendas and these did not necessarily address the hardships that families experienced. For example, the monthly cost of diapers was akin to the monthly cost of medicines – Rs 1800 – if only two diapers were used per day. The Khan family received free medicines for Omar from ARDSI-DC, but struggled to buy diapers and often purchased them on credit. With little positive effect and multiple side effects, Omar's medications were eventually stopped. The family then wanted the costs associated with free medicines (approximately Rs 2000 per month) to be transferred to subsidize the cost of his diapers. However, ARDSI-DC, fearing audit, refused. Their funders had donated money specifically for medicines and not diapers, even though the latter had equal, if not greater, utility to families.

The constant scramble of funds thus impinged on the capacity of the organization to broker a relationship between families and funders. Often the funders were privileged over the families. Quarterly newsletters that detailed ARDSI-DC's activities and the latest research and developments in dementia were mailed first to donors; if enough money was left over, then copies were sent to families. When ARDSI-DC commemorated its founder's day at an exclusive club, accolades and mementos were disbursed to management and patrons, but no carers or people living with dementia participated. For celebrations of World Alzheimer's Day in 2008, the names of all speakers were printed in the programme guide, except for the carers who were speaking; they were clustered as 'carers' under the heading 'caregivers' dilemma'.

These practices, neither novel nor unique to this organization, are symptomatic of the absurdities of aid flows and the pragmatic response from the sector. NGOs, like government bureaucracies, are political bodies with their own agendas, power elite, management problems, lack of sustainability, low replicability and minimal reach. The only difference, as Paul

Streeten has argued, is that 'NGOs may be doing less harm than governments in this field and may even be doing some good' (1997: 210).

Who Can Afford That?

Given the slow trickledown of funds, most families received little aid, cared alone and the majority privately bore the costs of care (n=13 out of 20). Only seven families received any formal assistance: three from the Central Government Health Scheme, which subsidized the cost of pharmaceutical drugs and medical treatments for these former employees of the state; and four from ARDSI-DC to purchase medicines. Of the families receiving aid from ARDSI-DC, two were lower middle class (the Khans and the Sadhwanis) and the other two were wealthier (Sen-Hamdari-Kaul and the Kochars). All had been referred for free medications following consultation at one of two ARDSI-DC memory clinics (OPDs in government hospitals). For a detailed account of the often chaotic and trying circumstances that was involved in obtaining such referrals, see chapters 2 and 3.

Further compounding the problem for families is the fact that public health expenditure in India is amongst the lowest in the world, at only 1.36 per cent GDP. Consequently, private spending is one of the highest worldwide with about 86 per cent of total health expenditure incurred privately and only about 31 per cent incurred by the public sector (World Bank 2013). Sickness and care are privatized and citizens mobilize their own resources, according to finances and levels of social support, to secure treatment. Among the twenty families, sources of income tended to coalesce into three overlapping categories: investments and savings (n=8), pensions from government and private industry (n=6 and n=5 respectively) and contributions from children (n=13). In line with the global gendered division of work into paid and unpaid forms, it is typically women who perform the latter and men the former; and women with dementia were more likely to rely on financial contributions from their family and personal savings (n=5 out of 8) while men also received a pension from former employers (n=8 out of 12).

Despite being middle class, many families struggled financially with the costs of care. Recurrent expenditures for allopathic medicines, diapers, a paid attendant and miscellaneous goods, such as cotton wool, talcum powder and condom catheters, were about Rs 11,000 per month (see Table 4.1). This figure excludes other ongoing costs for lost days of work, traditional and transcendental medicines, nutritional supplements, activities such as physiotherapy or doing yoga, transport to and from doctors'

TABLE 4.1 Costs of care for a person with dementia

Item	Rupees/month
Medicines	1,500.00[1]
Diapers	1,800.00[2]
Attendant	7,500.00[3]
Miscellaneous (Cotton wool, powder, condom catheter etc.)	500.00[4]
Total	11,300

Notes:
1. Calculation based on average cost as reported by ARDSI-DC.
2. Calculation based on Rs 30 per diaper with 2 diapers used per day, i.e. 60 diapers × 30 days.
3. Calculation based on agency rate of Rs 250 per 12 hour shift, i.e., Rs 250 per shift × 30 days.
4. Approximate costs.

consultations and doctors' fees. Also absent are non-recurring costs that families might incur for medical tests, health procedures and care equipment (e.g., rubber sheets and wheelchairs). At Rs 11,000 per month[2] (approximately A$199), the costs delineated above are incomplete and the whole picture has not been captured.

It is impossible to gauge a mean cost of the expenses because these figures oscillated significantly depending on income, class, identity and the health needs of each individual. Suneeta Sadhwani (41), a single woman with no siblings, spent almost nothing caring for her father, Hari Prasad (74). They received free medicines from ARDSI-DC, could not afford to hire an attendant and because Hari was able to toilet himself, spent nothing on diapers. Father and daughter stayed together in their own small two-bedroom flat in west Delhi and lived off Hari's retirement pension. Suneeta supplemented this by tutoring neighbourhood school children and described her earnings as 'our pocket money for extra expenses'. They did not own a car or scooter and rarely went out to restaurants or bought luxury items. Suneeta's recreation included reading magazines that her friends gave her, watching television and crocheting. Thus, even though the Sadhwanis were lower middle class financially, the monetary costs of Hari's care were not onerous.

Conversely, Namita Sood, also a single woman, homeowner and teacher, came from a wealthy background, but struggled to make ends meet. With her younger sister, she had spent seven years caring for her mother in their family bungalow in south Delhi. The Sood sisters had leased the top floors of their property to bring in additional income, but still experienced financial strain as Namita had quit her job to care full-time and had hired a physiotherapist, masseuse and nurse attendant during the day and two nurses at night. The sisters spent between Rs 90,000 and Rs 1 lakh per month on their mother's care and to meet these expenses, eventually Namita returned to work part-time.

The contrast between these families illustrates the difficulties in measuring the monetary costs of carework. How does a poorer, more vulnerable family such as the Sadhwanis have fewer financial pressures than a wealthier one such as the Soods? While the obvious answer lies in the kinds of goods and services purchased (e.g., no attendant versus five paid staff), the links between consumption, identity and imagination are also relevant. It was not that poorer families did not have attendants and richer ones did; nearly all families had some level of paid assistance in their carework. The difference was in the scale of assistance sought. Nina's search for a cure for Karamjit exemplifies this:

> He had this stem cell medicine for which we went to Cologne [Germany]. We were there for nearly four to five days, although it only took 20 minutes one day and 20 minutes the other day. [The doctor] said, 'Don't expect wonders at all, it is not a magic formula'. I said, 'Look I cannot lose him, I have to get him well'. It was quite a packet of money – so what? You know the care that he is getting, nobody can get it. Why? Because daily I am spending between 500 to 600 Rupees.

Nina and Karamjit paid for their travel to Cologne, while their younger son paid for the stem cell treatment. Though Nina never disclosed the entire amount of this treatment, she intimated that it was thousands of Euros. The resources spent on this venture indicate Nina's quest for an *ilāj* and the consumption-identity correlation. In India, consumption has been described either as central to modern national identity (Breckenridge 1995; Fernandes 2006; Rajagopal 2001) or as the flamboyance and self-seclusion of a few in the face of the blatant impoverishment of many (Das 2001; Varma 1998).

For many middle-class Indians, consumption is understood in moral terms; van Wessel's (2004) ethnography in the north Indian city of Baroda found that consumption was defined in opposition to ideals of elder care, the joint family and community. However, in cases such as Nina's, consumption was explicitly linked to elder care, family and the community. It becomes another measure of *sevā*. A good carer was one who would consume health and care services in her pursuit of an *ilāj*. The only difference between poorer and richer families was the scale of their consumption as determined by their resources and imagination. When families consumed less than they should have, there were criticisms:

He [Karamjit] goes to the barber and I would put the exact amount of money in his pocket. He would bring it back. He would fight at the shop saying, 'No, I won't give you, I've already given you' and that chap would come here saying, 'I haven't got my money and he is creating a ruckus in my shop'. He said, 'Either please stop him or please explain to him'. So I explained to him: 'For a meagre 30 Rupees you are shaming me; that lady doesn't give him money and he only has so much. Do you realize that it is a shame on me and us that we are not paying 30 Rupees?' (*Nina Bhagat, 70*).

'If I Get Depressed, Who Will Handle Him?'

If the costs of care associated with goods and services are difficult to measure, then calculating the subjective costs to familial relations, carer's health and the personhood of the individual with dementia is nigh impossible. Objective costs may be boiled down to a monetary figure, but subjective costs are the small and large slights that people experience that cost them in dignity, emotional wellbeing and physical health. These may include the distress that carers such as Josie and Shafia felt when their marital relations fundamentally and irrevocably deteriorated, or the indignities the Singh family experienced when trying to get adequate service in a *sarkari* hospital, or the fraught terrain of failure that Tandon negotiated in all his endeavours to find a cure for Sheila. These slights may also be in the minutiae of everyday life, for instance, when Bhageshwari's mother could not remember her name despite her daughter's insistence that she could, or in K.P. Aggarwal's indifference to his wife, or when Nandini came home to find her father had fallen down under a tap in the bathroom and was waiting for her to pick him up. These are small, hidden stories about change, loss and sadness. Their costs to carers are both physical and emotional.

A large body of research exists on the impact of dementia on family carers. Caring for a person with dementia can be stressful and depressing, creating financial worries, loss of employment and family conflict.[3] Carers for people with dementia are twice as likely to have a common mental disorder (typically depression) compared to carers or co-residents of people with depression (Patel and Varghese 2004). Qualitative work from rural Kerala ascertained that carers were usually educated middle-aged women who had been forced to either reduce or stop paid work in order to care – a decision that resulted in significant strain on the family budget. These women were also mothers and the work of caring for two generations left them tired, depressed and isolated. Many reported serious physical and psychological problems, managed through antidepressant medication, self-harm, or violence and abuse towards and from the person with dementia. Exposed to aggression and violence, these women felt they deserved such abuse (Shaji et al. 2003).

Many of these factors were evident in the families with whom I worked, whose members all complained of exhaustion, frustration and pain. Carers had health concerns – heart problems, cataracts, hip pain, back pain, Parkinson's disease, cancer and hyperthyroidism. Whether these were the end results of particular lifestyles (work stress, poor diet and lack of exercise), the by-products of age, the costs of caring, or unexplained acts of the universe, was irrelevant to them. While carers might develop theories for the cause of their loved one's dementia, they rarely speculated about the causes of their own health problems. For them, the assumption of the 'carer' role meant that they were to be supportive of the 'sick role' of the person with dementia. Most felt they must be stalwarts of care, irrespective of the costs to them. For them, illness was a luxury they could not afford:

> It [depression] happens but I cope with it myself. I do something or the other to keep myself busy. I watch TV or whatever talents I have in my hands I use them. Because if I become depressed myself, who will handle him? (*Suneeta Sadhwani, 41*).

> Whatever has to be done has to be done. *Baas* [that's it]. As long as we're here, as long as there's *sā:s* [breath], there's *a:ya:s* [effort]. My only prayer is that my *hāth-pair* [hands and feet] keep working because if my *hāth-pair* don't, then who will do this work? (*Sita Aggarwal, 63*).

Sita defined her capacity to care for her husband in terms of her working hands and feet. She had back pain, hip pain and leg pain and had been advised by her doctor not to bend much. But she soldiered on. As she described caring for her husband, K.P., her life seemed to transpire at a subterranean level: K.P. slept on a high bed with three mattresses, while she had a skinny mattress on the floor; when she prayed during her *puja* she knelt on the floor and bowed; and when I interviewed her, I sat on her living room sofa while she perched on a low stool. Her dedication to caring for K.P. was anchored in her own working body, in her muscles and her bones. Four times in a forty-five-minute recorded interview, she emphasized her desire for her hands and feet to work, 'I just pray, "Hai Bhaghvan [Oh God], let my *hāth-pair* work so I can lift him up."'

A productive body, defined through working hands and feet, is widely invoked in India in conjunction with ageing bodies. Old age or *buddhāpan* entailed a social reorganization of power relations wherein older people relinquished their roles within the household and younger members assumed greater responsibility through the provision of *sevā*. This restructure is based on the recognition of the bodily changes associated with age, described in the literature as *kāmzori* (weakness) and a failure of one's *hāth-pair* (Cohen 1998; Lamb 2000; Vatuk 1990). Cohen (1998) argued that when an older person's hands and feet stopped working, they were considered to be incoherent and unproductive. But Sita's distress was rooted in K.P.'s silence. It was not that K.P. could not talk; it was that he did not and was totally indifferent to her ministrations: 'I can just keep talking and get no answer so I [snap. She clicks her fingers]. I'm like a dog that just keeps barking and barking. I can keep crying, he'll say nothing, I can laugh, he'll say nothing, I can say, "I'm going" or "I'm not going," and he'll say nothing. He doesn't say anything'.

If silence and a loss of engagement were part of loss and degeneration, then the costs associated with these symptoms were transferred onto carers' bodies and expressed through the language of pain. Leg pain was frequently mentioned and described as swelling in the legs, dry skin and pain in the outer thigh area. When I asked Shivbaksh Chand how his health was, he said he had become very weak and lifted his *dhoti* all the way to his mid-thigh to show me one long skinny brown leg. Similarly, when I visited the Chopra family, Rubina, the daughter-in-law, said she experienced terrible pain in her legs that affected how many times she could climb up and down stairs. Suneeta Sadhwani said her legs felt 'weak,' but that her health was otherwise fine.

This weakness in your legs, can you describe it?
It's like an exhaustion. It feels like my legs are going to break, that I need to take some rest. I feel very tired sometimes, like as though there is no life in me.
To keep going?
Haa, but then I force myself to do it. But sometimes if I could just rest for a little while, if I could just rest, then it will be alright. It's not like my health is very down or anything like that.

Enough evidence has accumulated to demonstrate that psychological symptoms of distress may be somatized in the body as physical aches and pains with symptoms and experiences varying according to local contexts (see Kirmayer and Young 1998; Kleinman and Good 1985). In India, 51 per cent of all somatic complaints fit within the diagnostic criteria of common mental disorders (Patel et al. 1998). Depression especially tends to elicit somatic complaints, primarily from women. Body aches, autonomic symptoms, gynaecological symptoms, sleep problems, 'weakness' and tiredness are ubiquitous in clinical consultations (Pereira et al. 2007). But the leg pain that these carers cited bears further scrutiny – why leg pain? Why not pain in the hands or backs or wrists, which are also body parts that can experience strain as a result of caring?

Leg pain sits in an ambivalent juncture of culture, medicine, bodily disruption, ageing and loss. While it may be a culturally appropriate idiom for clinical depression and a physical manifestation of the psychological toll of confronting degeneration and loss on a day-to-day basis, the inverse is just as applicable. Leg pain may be just that – a pain in the legs that is a result of the physical stressors associated with caring. Instead of a confrontation with the bodily degeneration of the person with dementia, it may be a confrontation of the ageing of one's own body. Most carers were women in their fifties trying to manage men in their seventies and the physical labour necessary for such care is demanding. Caring includes manual handling and heavy lifting, cooking and cleaning and dealing with institutions and bureaucracies in hospitals, banks and NGOs, in heat and cold, through dust and fog, in the crush of people, money, family and social commitments. The work is not frenetic but constant, rolling in peaks and troughs as the days, weeks, months and years pass by. Such work will take its toll on the body.

For carers, leg pain becomes a way to stake a claim to the 'sick' role without the loss of power that such a position entails. Carers' identities are reshaped by the illness of another, who by virtue of being sick is unable to fulfil his or her social roles. If the person with dementia's *hāth-pair* no longer work, then the carers' hands and feet must now work for two. Multiple responsibilities must be fulfilled and carers get tired. Leg pain is a temporary means of claiming the debility of non-working *hāth-pair* without the associated loss of power and voice. As Suneeta said, 'It feels like my legs are going to break, but it's not like my health is very down or anything like that'.

Breakages and Cost

But low points in health do happen. In the literature, this is described as the 'breaking point' for carers; in Western nations it is typically at this juncture that the person with dementia is institutionalized. Factors contributing to institutionalization are severe cognitive, functional and behavioural disturbances as the dementia advances, combined with physical, psychological, emotional, social and financial stressors for his/her primary carer and little personal and social support from extended family, friends and the community (Banerjee et al. 2003; Hebert et al. 2001; Luppa et al. 2008).

A systematic review of dementia research undertaken in the US, Europe, Australia and Canada found that institutionalization is detrimental to people with dementia, their carers and national budgets (Luppa et al. 2008). In aged care facilities, people with dementia tend to deteriorate faster, their carers' decision to admit them is fraught with feelings of guilt, sadness and failure and governments worry about the burgeoning costs of institutionalization. Consequently, there has been a strong policy push, within these countries and in India, for dementia care to occur within the home and to be undertaken by unpaid carers, usually family members, with secondary support from governments, NGOs and paid attendants (Luppa et al. 2008). Accordingly, numerous initiatives have been developed. In countries such as Australia, these include short-term respite care, financial assistance, legal advice, support groups, day-care centres, home visits by social workers, volunteers and nurses and programmes such as art, gardening and music that the carer and the person with dementia can enjoy together. In India, short-term respite care, day-care programmes and home care attendants are most common.

Previously, in analysing legislative and policy documents, I illustrated that dementia care in India has been privatized and that people are denied access to institutionalized forms of care by the state (see Brijnath 2008). People with dementia are also largely excluded from private aged care facilities as the general admission criteria is that a client, described as an 'inmate,' must be physically and mentally competent (Patel and Prince 2001; Lamb 2009). This goes to the heart of access and citizenship, where those most vulnerable and least able to advocate for themselves, are denied care by the state and private institutions (Lamb 2009). As a result of this 'catch 22 situation', people with dementia can either be cared for by their families or, if they are alone (for whatever reason), face either the street or confinement in a state psychiatric facility. Drawing on research conducted in Goa (Prince and Trebilco 2005), I concluded that alongside the privatization of care, there was a lack of systemic support for families.

But many Indian families experience profound ambivalence about admitting a relative into any kind of a facility (Lamb 2009), an issue that is missing from my earlier work and that requires further inquiry. Less than 2 per cent of Delhi's older populations live in old age homes (Government of National Capital Territory of Delhi 2006); nationally the average is 2.73 per cent (Jamuna 2003). Even in Western nations, elder care occurs within the home[4] – in Australia, only around 6 per cent of older people are in aged care facilities (ABS 2013) and in the US it is around 5 per cent (Federal Interagency Forum on Aging-Related Statistics 2012).

In the study sample, almost all the families abhorred institutionalized care. Nina Bhagat described aged care facilities as a 'jail', Radha Menon broke off friendships when her friends suggested 'rehabilitation' for her husband and most carers seemed appalled by the notion of admitting their relative into any facility. Their feelings were based on an idealization of family and *sevā* and the horror of India's psychiatric institutions (where people with dementia might be institutionalized) (Pinto 2009, 2011). Institutionalization was a sign that a relative had 'gone mental' and to have a relative admitted into such a place was a sign of deep distress in the family.

It would not be hyperbolic to characterize long-term government psychiatric institutions in India as terrible places. Dank, harsh, prison-like and with appalling human rights records, such facilities reflect the worst aspects of colonial psychiatry and incarceration of the ill (National Human Rights Commission of India 1999). Given the negativity they elicit from nearly all sections of society, none of the relatively affluent middle-class families with which I worked had any direct dealings with them – except for one outlier – Josie.

Josie's story is harrowing and well-rehearsed. On the two separate occasions I heard this account, the narratives were near identical. The question is not of truthfulness, but of catharsis. Through repeat narrations of the story using the same words, Josie managed to infuse drama into the tale and simultaneously distance herself from the experience. Like Josie, I have found myself telling this story again and again, using her language and voice. It is neither easily told nor readily forgotten; the emotions it invokes make analysis particularly difficult as anthropology has not yet developed a language sophisticated enough 'to subject emotions (i.e. the wild) to analysis (i.e. rational civilization) without them losing their specificity as emotional "wilderness"' (Hage 2009: 77). I cannot claim in the accompanying analysis to have civilized this narrative – indeed, I too am lost in the emotional wilderness of this story and have not yet found my way to a rational shore.

'Mrs Singh, Think Twice Before You Bring Him Here'

On a baking April afternoon we sat on her living room floor where it was coolest. The fan swung furiously overhead and the tape recorder was switched on. Glasses of water rested on our sides. Josie, tall and slim, with short curly grey hair and a lilting voice, spoke in English:

> There was this doctor who approached the Alzheimer's Association and said, 'Look, mine is the only home which has a space for Alzheimer's patients. We have all the facilities, trained attendants, we do a jolly good job, it's clean and hygienic'. So I approached him because at that time it was going from bad to worse. I said to myself, 'Never again will I keep him in this house, never again, it's my life' – suddenly that surge of hate – 'That man [Su] is awful'. And I remember going to the doctor and he said, 'Mrs Singh, think twice

before you bring him here,' and I said, 'Doctor, I have made my decision, he has to go,' because the kind of physical violence was so frightening that the maid just took off from the house. He was like a demented caged animal. There were times that my entire head was swollen and it was tender for days and painful to the touch. My arm was sore because I was hurled against the panel and I don't even know when my nose was broken because my arm was raised and I had hit my head on the wall.

He [doctor] said, 'Look, since it's for you and you are an army wife, I will give it to you for Rs 35,000 but for the rest it is Rs 50,000'. I said 'Ok, anything for my sanity'. I worked round the clock, gave more tuitions to keep it going. It was a home for psychiatric patients, schizophrenics, drug addicts, alcoholics and patients with other mental disorders, all put together. They were almost in a cage. You could not talk to your patient. You had to talk to him through a glass window. And then I put my foot down and I said, 'Sorry! An Alzheimer's patient needs interaction. I have not put him here because I want to dump him. I've put him here because I am scared'. It was because of this violence that I kept going from one doctor to the other doctor, from this hospital to that hospital.

The first day when we went to leave him there, it was one of the most terrifying days of my life. He screamed and he ran amuck because he knew he was being put into a hospital. They strapped him down. He whacked them, they whacked him back. And then they just injected him when he was strapped. The next day he was like a zombie and for the next three days they just drugged him. He lost all his sense of bearing, but I think that is the breaking into [integration into] the hospital for all patients because for alcoholics and drug addicts, the withdrawal symptoms can be very severe. So they did the same thing to him to break him in. But every time I saw him, I remember, it was heartbreaking. I could only see him on a Sunday because apparently it would upset the routine of the others. That's what the doctor said to me and he took a down payment from me for two months because he knew I was a discerning woman, I would catch onto him.

Apparently when he used to pass potty, they used to wash him down with a hosepipe and the hose with water used to have bits of sand in it. He used to scream in pain. Imagine if you are being washed down with a hosepipe and you have these particles in the water, because it was ground water, hitting you. There were wounds all over his body and I used to ask the doctor, 'Why are there wounds?' and he would say, 'Oh, it is part of the disease'. I accepted it because then I did not know what Alzheimer's was like. It is only now that I realize that he was being physically attacked. If he ever turned violent, they used to physically handle him. I told you about the lacerations all over his bottom, having the mug hit him, it was the back edge of the mug hitting his tender skin and there were wounds. I used to ask the doctor, 'Why are there wounds on him?' and he said, 'Oh ma'am he wriggles in bed'. I said, 'If he wriggles in bed then all the skin should have peeled off his back'. He said, 'No! Mrs Singh don't ask us such questions, we're doing our best'. But I feel that these homes have to be questioned because his attendants were awful. Dirty, filthy, uneducated people, picked up straight from the road and dumped in there, given Rs 2,000 [per month] with food and told, 'Look after them'. They messed up his pants. They used to keep it [dirty pants] on till night and as a result he developed a severe fungal infection in his groin. It took me a good 20 days to one month to just de-infest him. Round the clock we gave him massages so as to bring him to some amount of normalcy.

I needed to write about it but I thought that it would have been very ruthless on my part to write about the doctor and his home as he came to my aid. And the second time again, when the violence continued. He was there altogether for almost six months, but staggered. First, for two months when he turned very violent. It was heartbreaking and the emotions are still there. Whenever I was leaving, I used to hug him and kiss him because that was all I could give him and one day he said, 'Come back, come back. Take me with you'.

[She weeps]

'Take me back, just take me back'. Now I wish I had taken him back, I could have been with him, but then I couldn't.

[Weeping]

But I tell you Bianca, each day he was in the hospital, I used to go through torture. I wish I could explain it to you – it doesn't give the caregiver any solace to send away your loved one, especially if you cannot share these moments together. It doesn't give you any solace. It tears you apart because you cannot turn a deaf ear, a blind eye, you cannot close your heart. Here is a man who needs you but, because you are helpless, you cannot do anything for him. It burns you each day.

The Institutional Costs of Care

At the heart of Josie's disturbing story is a complex relationship between exchange, cost and identity. Exchange here is monetary, reciprocal and redistributive (Polanyi 1957); Josie paid the doctor, he came to her aid and she handed Su's care over to paid attendants because of his violence. In these exchanges, the costs she incurred were financial and emotional. She broke Su's financial bonds, spent his pension and gave extra tuitions to pay the Rs 35,000 per month. As an objective cost and a high monetary sum, nevertheless it faded in comparison to the subjective costs that Josie paid. Su's admission into the facility, Josie's realization of the kind of care he received, his discharge and subsequent readmission and his final release when he returned home, was a process through which Josie's own sense of identity changed. She experienced and acknowledged her own failings, depression, rage and guilt, what Nussbaum has called 'shame and its relatives' (2004: 206).

Guilt and shame are to be distinguished here. The former is a type of self-punishment, anger at being unable to cope, whereas shame is self-flagellation through a focus on one's imperfections and defects. Guilt is action oriented, it is the feeling of being helpless or inadequate in doing something, but shame is an existential examination of one's own integrity and capacity (Nussbaum 2004). Josie experienced guilt but not shame about what happened to Su. She described feeling 'helpless' and 'burned'; unable to be with her husband even though she wanted to, her feelings of guilt lingered. But she was never ashamed of her decision, explaining, 'Here was a man who needed my complete attention but, because I had no choice, I was stuck with feeling guilty'.

Exploitation, so cutting within this story, was neither just the economic exploitation of Josie by the doctor nor the abuse of Su by the attendants in the facility – though both stand out vividly. There were also underlying class inequities. In the outsourcing of care to poorer people, whether at home, when the maid was there, or in an institution to untrained attendants, the reassignment of labour tells a broader story of who does what work, when and how and the deprivations that underpin these interactions.

The chronic shortage of resources and a trained mental health workforce has been well documented in India, as have the tatters of India's mental health system (Goel et al. 2004). The use of untrained, unqualified, poor people as attendants, while a substitute for this labour deficit, creates the conditions of abuse and violation because these attendants are deployed within institutional settings that are built on and continue to perpetuate the worst of biomedicine's historical treatment of the mentally ill (see Berrios and Porter 1995; Gilman 1996; Scull 1993; Shorter 1997). The results, as shown by Su's experiences, are disastrous for patients. It is more that madness is created than mental illness is treated. Institutionalization and exploitation of attendants also occur; they were paid Rs 2,000 a month, according to Josie, while the doctor, to whom she complained, charged her Rs 35,000 a month and instructed her not to ask questions.

The hierarchies within healthcare as shaped by class are also visible. Health is stratified both in doctor-patient relations (see chapter 3) and between health workers. Healthcare providers are keenly aware of each other and their status, as determined by their claim to knowledge, skills, salary and capacity to wield real and symbolic power (Nichter 1986). Banerji has been particularly scathing of the exploitative power of health practitioners:

> It is now being gradually realized that, in addition to being used as an instrument for alleviation of the suffering caused by diseases in individuals and in communities, health services have also been used as a political device to

increase dependence for exploitation of one class by another and to promote certain vested market interests (1978: 924).

The task, as Banerji (1978) points out, is to identify and alleviate such exploitation. Josie's story, pitched at the angry red of the spectrum, is an obvious and terrible case. Within the walls of a psychiatric institution, with its miseries and abuses, the objective and subjective costs are readily identifiable. Less straightforward are the exchanges between Josie, the doctor, the attendants and the transformations in Josie's identity. It is in these ambiguous zones that the boundaries are blurred. To try and clarify the links between exploitation, exchange and cost benefit – and even the applicability of such language – I move now from the micro to the macro and examine how they are operationalized in the pharma-economy of dementia care.

Pharma-economies of Care

Three factors affect production, distribution and consumption in the Indian pharmaceutical setting: (1) the commoditization of health goods and services within a pluralist health system; (2) the meta-medical meanings associated with health products; and (3) the impact of health policy on the profitability and hence production and distribution of medicines (Nichter 1996b).

Considerable work has been undertaken in the anthropology of pharmaceutical practices in areas of 'irrational' drug use, self-medication, pharmacy based practices, citizenship and the marketing of allopathic and *Āyurvedic* drugs.[5] Pills, potions and tonics from biomedicine and traditional medicine are widely available as discrete concoctions and in multiple combinations. About 70,000 kinds of drugs are estimated to be available in the Indian market, a figure 200 times greater than the 350 drugs listed on the WHO Essential Drugs List (Patel et al. 2005). This proliferation is especially remarkable because of the short history of the drug market in India; though production and marketing commenced in the nineteenth century, it was only in the post-independence period that this pharma-economy significantly expanded (Leslie 1989).

The pharmaceutical industry is extremely profitable in India because the notion of an *ilāj* is conflated with drugs. This is part of schismogenesis, a cyclical process whereby the medicalization of a problem increases demand for drugs, drives supply up and causes more medicines to flood the market. The greater availability and visibility of these medicines in turn raises consciousness about the problem and further exacerbates demand (Nichter and Vuckovic 1994). As a case in point, the social sign of ageing – *kāmzori* (weakness) – has been medicalized and there is an increased expectation amongst some middle-class older people that drugs can cure or reverse this symptom. Eighty-eight-year-old Kundan Lal Chopra felt he was less energetic than he used to be and took medicines for his blood pressure, nerves, depression, bones and breathing in a bid to cure his *kāmzori*. Still not satisfied, he sought further medical advice:

> I went to a private hospital, I saw a surgeon, I did an ultrasound [and] the doctor said, 'Who said to do all this?' I explained it all and he said, 'Weakness happens'. I said, 'Give me something for it'. Finally the doctor told me, 'The weakness you feel is because of age'.

Chopra's constant demand for medicines and search for an *ilāj* reflects the power located in medicines, the hope that doctors can give patients through drug prescriptions and the pervasiveness of drug taking in India. Such beliefs and practices are aided by a political economy in which the government has actively courted private investment in healthcare. Providing tax incentives (low to no tax), transferring the administration of healthcare centres to NGOs, subcontracting auxiliary services such as cleaning and catering in public hospitals, allotting land to build private facilities and offering low import duties on equipment and parts for diagnostic technologies (such as MRIs, CT scanners and x-ray) are just some of the strategies (Purohit 2001).

For their part, the private sector has embraced India's health markets. Foreign investment in the pharmaceutical sector has seen an annual growth of 20–25 per cent and in 2011 the pharmaceutical retail market was estimated to be worth Rs 432 billion ('Pharmacy Retailing to Grow Exponentially if FDI Norms Eased', 2009; Netscribes 2009). Sub-speciality hospitals and pharmaceutical chains have been established by corporations across India's megacities with plans to expand into smaller cities and towns. Private health insurance is booming; between 2006 and 2007 there was about 98 per cent real growth and in 2008, the insurance market was estimated to be worth approximately US$42 billion (USAID 2008). Within this lucrative political economy, supported by government and private investment, characteristics of India's health system, such as medical pluralism, doctor shopping and the deliverance of hope through a pharmaceutical *ilāj*, also acquire a commercial overlay and are informed by the distribution and division of resources in urban-rural areas and among the rich and poor.

In India, drug companies of varying scopes and sizes rigorously compete to promote their products. As has been noted in other countries, doctors are encouraged to increase prescriptions in exchange for gifts and favours (see Carpenter et al. 1996; Oldani 2004; van der Geest and Whyte 1988). Such practices can result in over-prescriptions (polypharmacy) and incompatible drug combinations, termed 'irrational' drug use (Linden et al. 1999; Sarkar 2004; Srinivasan 2004). 'Irrational' drug use also refers to the frequency and dangers of the popular practice of self-medication (Deshpande and Tiwari 1997; Greenhalgh 1987; Sarkar 2004). Drug resistance and widespread need to use more powerful medications is believed to be caused by irrational drug use (WHO 2009).

However, the term 'irrational' fails to capture the logic of practice by stakeholders in specific times and spaces. Pharma-economies are characterized by complex chains of relations between patients, doctors, pharmaceutical companies and pharmacists (Kamat and Nichter 1998). These relations are governed by claims to different kinds of capital – social, cultural, financial and symbolic – that are hierarchically structured and change according to settings. The order of these capitals is contingent on social relations rather than on economic criteria. Through a set of bodily and social practices, agents enact their claims to particular kinds of capitals, reinforce existing modes of domination and create specific and temporal logics of practice (Bourdieu 1990). The centrality of doctors in OPDs, for example, was based on the privileging of knowledge and symbolic capital as evinced in doctors' capacity to read scans, diagnose disease and prescribe medicines. All other players in the OPD accepted this power of doctors and adjusted their behaviour accordingly. But in other settings where the power of the doctor was diminished, people's behaviour towards doctors also changed. At ARDSI-DC functions, for instance, doctors' praise for the NGO's services were used to produce the social capital necessary to garner more support from policy makers and funders. In these settings, the NGO, not the doctors, took centre stage.

But in *sarkari* OPDs, the doctor was omniscient and patients, families, attendants, medical students and administrative staff played their roles in establishing this power hierarchy. This authority, rooted in knowledge and symbolic capital, also had an economic base. To understand this economic chain of relations, it is necessary to introduce one more set of actors into the OPD milieu – the representatives from pharmaceutical companies who are colloquially known as 'med reps'.

The practices in which med reps and doctors engaged differed according to hospital, doctors and settings. In Yashaswini's OPD, med reps were rare and never stayed long. The observations I describe below are from another *sarkari* hospital called 'Cornwall'. The Cornwall Hospital has colonial roots and dated facilities against which the present enormity of patient demand is a stark contrast. In this hospital's OPD, four to five doctors clustered round a desk for two hours, while 100–200 patients would arrive mainly for prescription refills (no more than about 20 per cent of the presentations were new cases). Like in Yashaswini's OPD, epilepsy was the most common cause of presentation, followed by headaches, psychosomatic complaints and neurological concerns in which dementias were classified. The chronicity of such diseases and the prescription refills that their management necessitated made the Cornwall OPD particularly attractive to med reps.

On average five med reps – sent by subsidiaries of companies such as Ranbaxy® and Pfizer® – were present throughout the consultations. They distinguished themselves from doctors and patients through their embodiment of financial affluence. Unlike patients who dressed in bright colours and doctors who wore white laboratory coats, med reps were always formally attired in sober colours, with polished shoes and the latest mobile phones clasped at their belts. Their expensive colognes contrasted with the dusty, sweaty odours that emanated from everyone else. This image itself is a dated cliché; Kamat and Nichter (1997) made remarkably similar observations over ten years ago about Mumbai's med reps. Like the med reps in their study, most med reps here were also men (only once did a young woman come from a pharmaceutical company) and held degrees in general science, rather than clinical qualifications. These men presented themselves as young, gauche and uncertain and always seceded to the doctors' authority. Although the med rep's behaviour changed according to the doctor's age, sex, qualifications, experience and speciality (for an alternative account see Kamat and Nichter 1997), in the Cornwall OPD, with its neurology focus and specialist senior doctors who were predominantly men, med reps were always deferential. They seldom approached clinicians in the OPD and instead would stand in a corner of the room while the doctors sat in the middle. Aside from marketing, they also managed patient flow, organized patient files and bought coffee and cold drinks for doctors when required.

Med reps disliked being referred to as such and preferred the label 'product executive'. While I have used the term 'med rep' for expediency, it is uncomplimentary and obfuscates another layer of marketers – the *test-wallahs*. These are agents employed by local private pathology and neuroimaging centres to market to doctors and patients. When a doctor prescribed an MRI scan, he could either recommend the *test-wallah* to the patient or the *test-wallah* would approach the patient directly and hand over his business card.

A hierarchy exists between med reps and *test-wallahs*. The former were contemptuous of the latter because of the percentage of profits that *test-wallahs* shared with doctors. Med reps gave up to 20 per cent of their earnings from each OPD session to the doctor, but *test-wallahs* from smaller and more precarious businesses could offer 30 to 40 per cent. This was according to Nitin, a cheerful and forthcoming senior med rep, supervising a number of 'field boys'. His job was to court doctors in Delhi's hospitals to prescribe his company's medications. *Sarkari* hospitals were preferred over private facilities because the high volume of patients netted bigger profits and a large drug company could earn about Rs 80,000 worth of business per OPD session.[6]

For doctors, the profit margins were generous and they could earn between Rs 20,000 and Rs 150,000 per month from drug companies. However, to maintain the hierarchy of capital, the doctor's authority and to avoid the stain of medicine for money, an etiquette had developed around 'gifts'. Doctors could ask for expensive medical textbooks, conference funds and overseas trips for their families instead of and in addition to money. Even when money was to be given, discretion was paramount and cheques were preferred over cash. These could be slipped into one of the many product reports that med reps were continuously giving to doctors. As Nitin explained to me: '*Arre* madam there are hundreds of ways to do *juga:r* [manoeuvrings]. Each of these doctors has ten, ten relatives. Some of the cheques are in daughters' names, wife's name, mother's name and the accounts are then all linked'.

Giving gifts to doctors is commonplace in India and the pharmaceutical industry is a relatively new player. Cooperation, flattery and gifting are practices that patients and families have used to personalize their relationship with doctors, to improve the quality of their treatment and to make bribes in order to secure speedier services (Jeffery 1988). These practices are located in the historic doctor-patient relationship where giving a gift, in addition to commercial exchange, invoked a bond of moral reciprocity between the doctor and patient. Mauss wrote of the etiquette of gifting in India:

> Contracts, alliances, the passing on of goods, the bonds created by these goods passing between those giving and receiving – this form of economic morality takes account of all this. The nature and intentions of the contracting parties, the nature of the thing given, are all indivisible (1923, 1966: 77).

In *sarkari* hospitals where gifting is illegal, one source of doctor's income has thus been eliminated. Doctors cannot, and in my observations did not, charge their patients fees. In the context of their working lives, long hours and patient demands, their salaries were meagre; a junior doctor could expect to earn Rs 25,000 and a senior consultant Rs 50,000 per month. For these doctors, 'gifts' from pharmaceuticals were important sources of income and prestige. This is not to say that all doctors accepted 'gifts' or asked for money; some had refused such overtures and med reps steered clear of them.

Within this complex pharma-economy of care, drugs represent the Janus face of cost and benefit. Costs, both objective and subjective, are incurred by people with dementia who experience the side effects of drugs, their families who manage these side effects, the NGO that may subsidize the cost of drugs, the doctors who might compromise their clinical standards through over-prescription for commercial gain and the pharmaceutical companies and med reps who pay kickbacks to the doctors for such prescriptions. But benefit may also be present in the alleviation of distressing symptoms for the person with dementia, the comfort families derive in knowing they are trying every *ilāj* possible, the funding that NGOs garner to continue delivering services, the hope that doctors are able to provide through prescriptions and the possibility that the pill, which pharmaceutical research has developed, does mitigate against distressing symptoms.

Ultimately it is neither theoretically useful to situate doctors at the polarities of corruption and sanctity nor practical to call for an end to gifting – the phenomenon is global. Both positions disregard the economic and working lives of *sarkari* doctors as well as the sociality of a gift in India. And if health and care have moral, political and social meanings, which are articulated in the materiality of everyday relations between doctors, patients, families and med reps, then it is more productive to focus on the microeconomic realities of these interactions and ask, as Mark Nichter has done, 'Rational for who and rational in what contexts?' (1996a: 252).

Domestic Economies

Nowhere perhaps are the ambiguities of care rendered more obvious than within the home, when paid attendants are hired to care. Within this space the complexities of exploitation, exchange and cost benefit come together to inform practices of identity and notions of family (see also Ray and Qayum 2009). Of the twenty families, nine had hired full-time attendants specifically to care for their relative with dementia and two had part-time assistance. The full-time attendants who lived with the families (n=3) were unmarried, in their early twenties and came from cities and villages elsewhere in India. In the remaining six cases, the full-time attendants worked shifts of ten to twelve hours, were married, in their mid-thirties and lived in Delhi with their families. Additionally, all families had servants who provided some secondary support by cooking, cleaning and washing. Five families could not afford to hire an attendant to care, while some hired attendants despite the financial stress this would create. Josie and Nandini, for instance, struggled with the costs of care but hired attendants so that they could remain employed and keep earning.

The decision to hire an attendant was largely based on household income and women's workloads. Women's labour encompassed paid and unpaid work. Women such as Vandhana, Sarojini and Bhageshwari were not employed, but hired attendants so as to manage their other responsibilities of housework and childcare. Such a market transfer of care is common among families in the region and beyond (Baldassar et al. 2007; Brijnath 2009; Hochschild 2000, 2003; Lan 2002; Srinivas 1995).

In all cases paid attendants were poor and had limited formal education. Attendants were distinguished from domestic servants by terminology, salary and care oriented tasks. The English word 'attendant' applied to those who were paid to undertake carework for people with dementia, while Hindi words such as *a:ya:* (maid) or *didi* (older sister) were used to refer to domestic servants. A live-in attendant could earn up to Rs 10,000 per month while a live-in servant earned up to Rs 4,000. Attendants focused on the physical and mental aspects of care for the person with dementia; servants were charged with overall housework and childcare. However, attendants could commence working in a household as a servant and then be asked to care for a person with dementia. Bhageshwari's maid was often asked to sleep in Bhageshwari's mother's room at night and to take her to the toilet, for which she was paid additional money. The oscillation between the category of 'maid' and 'attendant' illustrates the overlap in job roles and the similar class orientations of both groups. Attendants and servants were poor people with few opportunities.

At the request of a community health centre, ARDSI-DC trained women from a slum called 'Kamini', located on the north-east fringes of Delhi, to become paid attendants in families' homes (see Fig. 4.1). Kamini housed around 64,500 people over 200 acres. These residents were either displaced from the gentrified sanctums of inner-city Delhi during the Clean Delhi Drive initiative of the 1970s[7] or were impoverished villagers from the failing farmlands of neighbouring Uttar Pradesh. Kamini's women, in addition to seeking employment as attendants, were also domestic servants, makers of incense sticks, decorators of *bindis* and seamstresses. Their husbands were vegetable vendors, daily labourers and auto-rickshaw drivers. Their older daughters sometimes assisted them with housework and childcare; their sons might be rag pickers and rickshaw pullers. Kamini's residents, by virtue of their financial vulnerability, led more fragile lives and comprised part of the 53.1 million people (approximately 14 per cent of the total urban population) who live below the poverty line in India today (Government of India 2013).

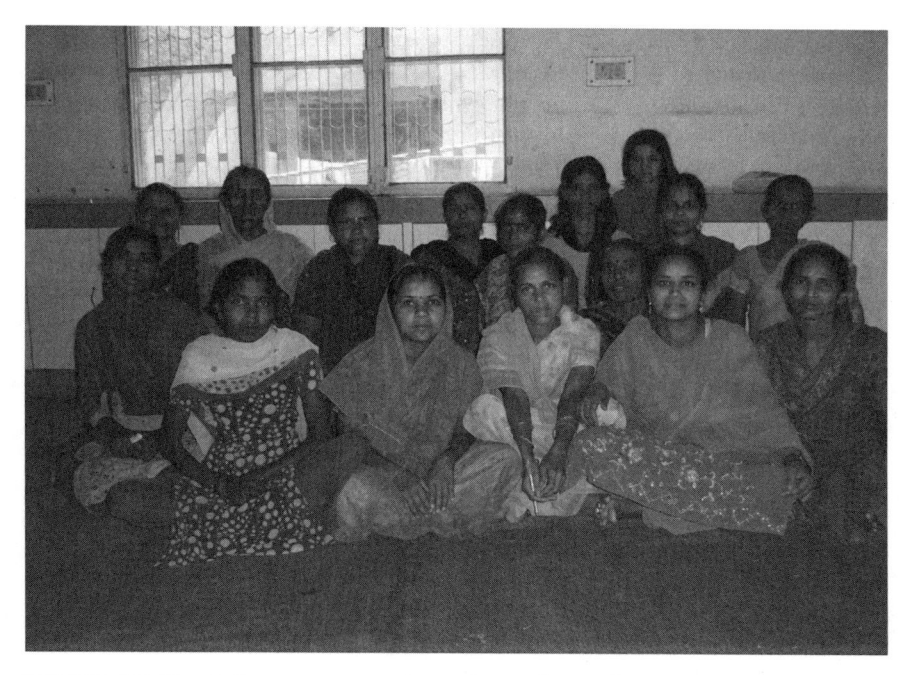

FIGURE 4.1 Kamini's women, training to be paid attendants

The disparity between attendants' background and those of the families for whom they worked created points of tension. While the families had money, purchasing power and plentiful choices of how to spend their Rupees, they also grappled with the consequences of the growing rift between the affluent and the poor, especially in urban settings. As Pavan Varma succinctly puts it, this is 'the middle class of a poor country' (1998: 172), where the walls between classes are stringently guarded and involve much more than just the denial of opportunities to the poor. The frustrations of inequality contributed to an increased sense of danger in everyday Delhi life and according to Inspector Tyagi, the main perpetrators of crimes against the aged in Delhi are their domestic servants: 'Robbery is the main motivation and in rare cases it is a crime of passion. There is invariably assault, battery, murder'. The Senior Citizen's Cell cautions, 'Don't allow servants to have access to your cupboards, safes etc' (Delhi Police Senior Citizen's Cell 2008).

The way in which families and attendants felt about each other was shaped by these wider forces of class and both parties resented their interdependency. Josie felt as if she was being held to 'ransom', Nandini described being 'rooked' (robbed) and Vandhana was determined not to be dependent on any paid carers. Such feelings are commonplace in master-servant relationships in India and are based on the instability of power relations between families and servants. Trawick wrote of an 'intuitive recognition of Sartre's dictum that in reality the master is the slave,' when she described her interactions with her Tamil family – 'Thus when I said to Anni that I felt she was treating me like a queen, she replied, "A queen has no freedom"' (1990a: 55).

Caste, in this context, was not explicitly articulated and discriminations based on 'untouchability' were largely absent. However, caste barriers were reinforced in other ways; traits such as thievery, laziness, ineptitude to learn new things and uncontrolled fertility were associated with attendants and domestic servants. Pinto (2004) made similar findings in rural north India and the Jefferys' have pithily noted that 'money itself discriminates' (2008: 61). Families' discontent was based on the high rate of absenteeism among attendants, the salaries they charged (Rs 250 to Rs 300 per shift) and their laxity with regard to activities such as bathing, toileting and mobility. Namita Sood, who had had relatively positive experiences, said:

> You know that whole business of coming for duty, not coming for duty, they had personal problems, they were not willing to learn new techniques . . . But when someone doesn't know what to do and is not willing to learn . . . We were very fortunate that for five years we had a team which was pretty well managed.

The Sood family were an anomaly because they recognized the demands caring could make on a single person and so opted for a team approach. Most families, unable to afford this, instead made heavy demands on individual attendants. Shifts were typically ten to twelve hours long, excluding commuting time to and from work, which could result in a fourteen to sixteen hour day. For example, the cheapest way to travel between Kamini and south Delhi (where the majority of families lived) was a two-hour bus ride each way. Many of Kamini's women could not manage such distances on a daily basis while meeting the needs of their own homes and children.

Some attendants tried to redress the barrier of geography by living with families. But this presented problems too as attendants were then available twenty-four hours a day. And if the distances of geography were difficult to deal with on a daily basis, then the barriers of inequity were near impassable. Attendants might have had their food, shelter and salary provided, but they did not eat with the family, or sleep in a room of their own, or wear similar clothes, or earn anything relatively proportional to what was sometimes asked of them. A small but telling example was the lack of surnames among attendants. Their names – Saroj, Sandra and Santosh

– contrasted with the names of the middle-class men whom they cared for – K.P. Aggarwal, A.P. Arora and S.T. Pillai. It was a standard practice that an older man's first name might be condensed into initials and only his last name retained while a poorer person's first name was retained and their surname forgotten.

However, attendants did have power and agency, which they exercised through strategies of reciprocity, redistribution and monetary exchange. None explicitly articulated such methods, but in the grumblings and disgruntlements of families, the forcible sharing of power can be seen. Families talked about attendants' expectation of gifts and bonuses in addition to salaries:

> It was Rs 5,000, then after a year we increased it, this year again we increased it. Like this we keep increasing it – Rs 500, Rs 500 and then Rs 300, Rs 300. Otherwise nothing would work. On his birthday I give them a gift, on their birthdays I give them gifts, I make a cake, like this, like this (*Shilpi Mukherjee, 72*).

> I got rooked badly. Initially I used to have this travelling job. They [attendants] come for two days and understand the entire vulnerability of this family. The first one I had, I used to get all these high protein diets for dad and she didn't give him any, she whacked it all off. No fruits being given. I mean these were two things where nutrition was concerned. So every time I would come back the doctor would have to be called in because he was very weak or he's got aggression (*Nandini Pillai, 52*).

Theft was used as a means of sharing value through the redistribution of goods. Again, attendants did not express this, but families complained of missing nutritional supplements, silver and cameras. Paradoxically these losses, while sustainable for families, were frowned upon but passively tolerated. Families, mired in relations of interdependency, had little choice but to accept such theft if they wanted to retain their attendant's services. This ran contrary to the Brahminical ideas of personal property and gifting, where property is assumed to be an extension of the self, to be given (rather than taken) to enrich others (Mauss 1923, 1990). Bhageshwari explained this contrary logic:

> What started happening was things started disappearing from the house – upstairs, downstairs – [in] both houses things started disappearing. I lost my silver from my kitchen, my sister lost her camera. So you have to be very careful. But then you can't keep a check on them every time . . . These women, they're having a tough time in life because they're also doing this work.

For attendants, the desire to be treated humanely and to receive adequate payment for their services was important. Saroj, from Kamini, stated:

> See we are poor people. We need enough security so that my husband and my children are [secure]. I should get enough salary so that the people at home can live on it and that it covers the rent and everything else. We give them so much help, we do so much for them, they should at least give us enough so that we can support our own homes and feed our children.

In addition to money, attendants also imbued in their work claims of kinship, reciprocity and *sevā*. People with dementia were often referred to as 'uncle', 'aunty', '*mātāji*' (mother) and '*papaji*' (father) rather than 'sir' or 'ma'am'. This signalled the attendants' respect for their employers and elders and simultaneously avoided the pitfalls of class and a detached employer-employee relationship (Vatuk 1969). Attendants explained their work as doing *sevā* for a parental figure and through their claims of kinship derived meaning from the work they performed. It was a way of trying to gain the 'attendant affection, rights and obligations' of other family members by providing care like family and doing what family does (Karner 1998: 70). Many had a deep love and affection for the people they cared for.

> I like doing this work. It is *sevā* for the old and elderly and in your own heart also you get a relief knowing that this person – who is like my mother – [that] her body is also working (*Saroj*).

> Work is work and everyone must find meaning in it. There is no such thing as *chhoṭa* [little] work or *baṛa:* [big] work. Doing work for the patient in their home, this is *sevā*, I'm doing *sevā* for a helpless person who can no longer do their own work (*Sandra*).

Claiming kinship, as daughters and nieces, enabled female attendants to overcome gender barriers. They could care for men and women, unlike male attendants who could only care for men. During fieldwork, the gender of paid attendants matched with the gender of people with dementia (male attendants=5; female attendants=4) but this was not always the case and many families reported hiring women to care for older male relatives.

Nevertheless, the strategy of fictive kinship, while an exercise of power and agency, was still made from a position of vulnerability. It was a double-edged claim for it also exposed many attendants to the risk of being exploited for additional kinds of unpaid labour (Lan 2002). Paying for care relieved the families' burden of care by relocating it onto poorer, more marginal bodies. Jahangir recalled: 'This has happened to women I know, where they go to do this work and the family is very nice to them, does a little *chamcha:giri* [flattery] and then they are doing all the work. This way our work just keeps increasing and increasing'.

Increased demands led to an escalation of physical and emotional stress and eventual fatigue and burnout. Many attendants resigned and sought work elsewhere. Even so, for some the bonds of kinship still held. Sandra, an attendant for seven years, recollected:

> That old lady died about two years ago. I could not go [to the funeral] because I was working [here]. But I would always call *bha:bhi* (sister-in-law, but here refers to Sandra's employer) and keep asking, 'How is ma's state? How is she?' Even though she gave me so much trouble I remember that family very fondly.

As Sandra's story illustrates, claims to kinship were rooted in the emotional work of caring and *sevā*. Even when attendants left their employ, such feelings governed their continued contact with previous employers. Those attendants who stayed and cared until the person with dementia died experienced a profound sense of loss. In addition to feelings of grief, they also had to confront the loss of employment and income. The death of the person also signified the demise of the reason that validated their claim to kinship. Relationships with families now changed and few could revert or become domestic servants within these households. Death also ironed out the ambiguities in power relations, for families could afford to dismiss attendants. But this was often a mutual dissolution and when attendants sought work elsewhere, families helped by seeking new employment for them, providing referrals and extra money for the transition.

Conclusion

Using three concepts – cost, identity and exchange – I have laid out the topography of the economy of dementia care in India. The space within these terms has been explored through their application in the broader social spaces of Delhi. I have discussed the home, the psychiatric institution, the OPD and the pharmaceutical industry, populated by families, people with dementia, attendants, doctors, med reps and NGO workers, in order to explain the complexity of this economy. I have moved beyond questions of affordability to try and capture the relationality and emotions that underpin these economic exchanges. Cost, as was shown, is associated with specific objects – drugs, diapers and catheters – and with hidden subjectivities, such as feelings of sadness, fatigue and guilt but also *sevā*, duty and reciprocity. What appears at first glance to be beneficial may have darker undertones; the price may be paid in intangible ways. Josie's admission of Su into a psychiatric facility because of his violence, families' hiring of attendants to help manage carework and doctors' prescriptions of medicine to give hope and relief, all have their accompanying shadows: Josie's guilt about how Su was treated, families' exploitation of attendants and doctors' acceptance of 'gifts' from pharmaceutical companies.

Identities within these exchanges are ambiguous, fluid and uncertain, but also (re)fashioned and cemented according to notions of care and love. Exploitation and agency, hope and despair, love and money, inform the commercialization of care through market exchanges, the reciprocity in giving and receiving gifts and the redistribution of power and materiality through the bonds of kinship. It is not that there are equal and opposite narratives for every story, but rather that across a landscape of inequity, at different points, people share, exploit, dominate, subjugate and are kind to each other. Using the same examples cited above – Josie, families and attendants, doctors and drugs – these factors are also evident.

In mapping such complexities of cost, exchange and identity, a balanced analysis is not possible. In the macro-economy of care, the gaps in service, the politics of delivery and the risks of outsourcing care are visible. When set within the larger picture of diagnosis and treatment, such costs seem wholly negative. This is not to deny the quiet satisfactions and joys of caring and these aspects will now be elucidated through an analysis of the role of food, *sevā* and love in daily life.

Notes

1. As of 17 December 2013, A$1= Rs 55.3.
2. In 2008 the average middle-class wage in Delhi was Rs 50,000 per month.
3. For research in India see: Dias et al. (2004), Emmatty et al. (2006), McCabe (2006), Patel and Prince (2001), Prince and Trebilco (2005), Shaji et al. (2003), The 10/66 Dementia Research Group (2004) and Varghese and Patel (2004). For work internationally see: Annerstedt et al. (2000), Braekhus et al. (1998), Brodaty and Green (2002) and Hux et al. (1998).
4. Notions of home differ considerably between India and Australia and between India and the US. In India, joint families are common with many generations living in the same property and sharing (theoretically if not always literally) income. In the US and Australia, children do not typically live with their ageing parents nor do they share finances.
5. For more on irrational drug use and self-medication see Deshpande and Tiwari (1997), Greenhalgh (1987) and Patel et al. (2005); for pharmaceutical practices see Kamat and Nichter (1997, 1998) and Nichter (1996a, 1996b); for the links between pharmaceuticals and citizenship see Ecks (2005); and for advertising

and marketing of allopathic and *Āyurvedic* drugs see Cohen (1998) and Langford (2002).
6. Each government hospital has about two to three neurology OPDs per week.
7. Clean Delhi Drives are a recurring event organized by the Delhi Government where, to make way for gentrification and purported new developments, people are moved out of their existing homes into resettlement colonies. Most often those moved are people who live in slums. These moves typically leave them worse off as they have fewer economic opportunities and have access to poorer infrastructure in their new fringe dwellings.

5. ALZHEIMER'S AND THE INDIAN APPETITE

BEGIN BY COMBINING MANY INGREDIENTS – memory and nostalgia (Appadurai 1988, 1996), kinship (Manderson 1986), relationality and pleasure (Mintz 1985), domestic citizenship (Das and Addlakha 2001) and the sensory experiences of ingestion, excretion and its management (Jackson 1989). Mix these ingredients in the body, making sure its orifices and pores are open to inclement weather: fingers should smart from crushing too much chilli into a bubbling vindaloo, the head should be numbed from drinking ice water on a 45 degree afternoon when the sweat trickles down knees and the mouth should pool with saliva when the sourness of pickled mango seeds are sucked stringy for the last vestiges of flavour. Embrace such a sensory anthropology: explore how taste, touch, sight, sound and smell affect physical and emotional health in people with dementia and their carers, how food invokes sensations of power, happiness and loss.

Take the body as the 'subject of culture ... the existential ground of culture' (Csordas 1990: 5), not just the mechanics of digestion. Tongue, taste buds, stomach and intestines are not just ways of processing food, but also the means by which food is felt and experienced. Tangy curry, pungent turmeric and crunchy red onions can turn rancid when absorbed and amalgamated into the body and gas, cramps and bloating alongside fullness, contentment and laziness are part of the degustatory experience. Eating is rooted in bodily processes of discomfort and pleasure. The fond remembrance of a meal lingers in the taste buds, the overeating of nostalgia lies in a full belly and the heartburn of an ageing body reflects chagrin for bodies that can no longer eat as they used to. These are also examples of how the medium of food can invoke memory and vitality against the loss associated with age and degeneration.

Ghar ka kha:na (home cooking) is used in this chapter to describe when the hearth and the home are not what they used to be and a nostalgic connection to the past is made through home-cooked meals and juxtaposed with contemporary family life and food purchased from outside. Food cooked within the home is part of the disciplinary project of care enacted both on the caregiver and the care receiver. For as long as the person with dementia eats, the work of surveillance, routine and containment is ongoing, threading discipline into kin relations within a wider social milieu and on the body and bodily processes. It is a relation of power and citizenship within the home (Das and Addlakha 2001), a status accorded to the carer and the person with dementia. But implicit in this disciplinary project, and undermining it, are memory and nostalgia. I distinguish them through taste: memories are tasteful and tasteless, bitter and sweet, whereas nostalgia is always sweetly melancholic. As the unspoken memories of loss, famine, deprivation and hunger, whether actually endured or collectively imagined, enter into the domestic sphere, anxieties ensue around hunger and wasting. Carers experience such emotions when the person with dementia stops eating – a point I return to later.

On assembling these ingredients, as yet raw and unassimilated, the recipe is as follows: first, introduce the links between food and Indian identities; then combine and complicate the relationship between food, *sevā*, discipline and domesticity; separate the health discourse imbued in it; discard the waste that is generated; and finally feast on the sweet pleasures of feeding.

Food and Identity

Gastropolitics in India has undergone a profound change in the last three decades, incorporating the long established moral and medical taxonomy of food into a more recent global gustatory landscape that focuses on consumption, identity and change. Traditionally, the organization of food and eating aligned with relations of class, caste and ageing, with attendant politics of purity and exchange. Food in India has had multiple meanings beyond mere sustenance; it extends to cultural, economic and legal claims of rights, responsibilities, complaints and conflicts as well as the structuring of caste-ordered substances (Khare 1998; Khare and Rao 1986; Marriott 1976; Smith 1990). Who can eat what, where, when and prepared by whom is determined by a complex capillary network that transcends discrete categories and roles of 'Brahmin priest', 'Kṣatriya warrior' or 'Shudra leatherworker' (Marriott 1976).

Marriott's work (1976) in particular highlighted that the transfer or exchange of food in trade, alms or feasts was also an exchange of bodily substance codes. If gifting in Hinduism was giving a part of oneself (Mauss

1923, 1966), then eating was the literal ingestion, absorption and amalgamation of that personhood. Within such a paradigm there were stringent boundaries around purity, pollution and dirt in food exchange. But as Appadurai (1981) points out, such rules were also a response to the homogenizing effects of food. Sharing a meal, eating together – mashing hot starchy rice between fingers, slurping yoghurt, commenting on the saltiness of a dish – invokes a deeper relationality beyond the parameters of polite conversation. Sharing food is a way of making memory and building social relations. When I went to interview Kundan Lal (K.L.) Chopra for the first time, his entire family was present and I was served breakfast, tea and two steaming *gobi-parathas*[1] slathered with *ghee*. Chintu, K.L.'s younger daughter-in-law, who made this meal, explained: 'I hardly get the chance to do this – we're all busy: I'm at work, with the children; my husband's in his shop, we're always busy. It's rare that we get to sit together and just have a chat. But whatever time we spend together we try to make it memorable.'

Food was critical to memory making, hospitality and the structure of all my interviews with families. Vandhana Arora and I met over her *pao-bha:ji*, *gula:b jammuns*,[2] grapes, tea and Limca®. Similarly, Suneeta Sadhwani and I ate *rajma-cha:val*[3] on her living room carpet after our second interview and Bhageshwari Srivastava offered me homemade chocolate cake while I interviewed her. But while eating was symbolic of my relations with families, tea had soaked into the foundations of my fieldwork. Tea was ubiquitous, drunk with key service providers and families, and to refuse an offer of tea was inconceivable:

> Do you want to drink tea?
> *No, no, it's ok. I have water [point to my bottle]*
> [Shocked] You don't drink tea?
> *[Placating] I do*
> [Decisively] Fine, then I'll make tea.

Cha:y, sweet, hot, silky, flavoured with green cardamom, boiled and boiled, often with milk skins floating on top, arrived during the course of the interview. I hate tea. But I quickly learned that drinking it proved less disruptive to the interview and with secret grimaces and a clenched stomach I swallowed it. *Cha:y* was a social lubricant, building mutual respect through the acceptance and ingestion of personhood and even in the Cornwall OPD, doctors would ensure that med reps brought tea for me. If my ethnography is about stories of care, then drinking *cha:y*, feeling the sugar widen my eyes and lift me from the lethargy of heat, was how I acquired the energy to listen.

But, to return to Appadurai's (1981) point of the homogenizing effects of food, eating together can also be dangerous because it can threaten existing social hierarchies. Rules around food preparation and consumption reflect the dangers of cooking and eating, for food is also associated with dirt, taboo and fears of the unknown outside the home. *Ghar ka kha:na* is as much about the nostalgia for a home-cooked meal as it is about the perceived excesses and impurities of restaurant and street preparations.

Concurrently, dirt in food is tacitly accepted and folded into dietary practices, often in the form of jokes. The health risks that arise from eating dirty food are often packaged as jocular warnings, a strategy that can be traced to colonial Anglo-Indian domestic home companions (Procida 2003). Food and dirt were and continue to be matched together. In colonial India, for example, English women were advised not to visit their kitchens for fear of the conditions under which their food was prepared by native cooks (Chattopadhyay 2002), just as in more contemporary times 'Delhi belly' is the expected consequence of eating Indian street food in the traveller blogosphere. There is little doubt of the unsanitary conditions in commercial kitchens and food prepared by street vendors – stale oil, bacteria rich water, simultaneous handling of raw and cooked meats, rats and roaches and the personal hygiene of cooks themselves – are gastronomic dangers that any eater of 'outside' food will confront in India.

However, the dangers of outside food also represent a more secular, anonymous exchange of marketplace and bodily substance codes. In not knowing who, how and under what circumstances food is prepared, eating out becomes an exchange of bodily substance codes across religions, caste, class and spatial barriers in exchange for money. Ironically, the affluent urban middle class within and outside India, powerful and with the most to lose within the class hierarchy, is the driving force behind this change. The Indian middle classes desire their own regional *ghar ka kha:na* – like Bengali *dum-alu*, Punjabi *parathas* and Tamilian *dosa* – alongside culinary exoticisms such as sushi, tacos and pasta (Srinivas 2007).

Transnationally, the availability of pre-packaged, popular nostalgic foods marketed 'as mother made it' in places such as Boston and Melbourne, but also Bangalore and Mumbai, strengthens links between homeland and diasporas (Srinivas 2006). Such foods and marketing techniques complicate geographies of home and abroad and rules around caste and class. Definitions of home-cooked and exotic meals are now so blurred that as Tulasi Srinivas writes, 'It would appear that authenticity is not questioned, as long as the copies that appear authentic are provided, as symbolic anchors on which identification can unfold' (2006: 207).

In short, the aspirational urban Indian and the nostalgic diaspora want their cake and to eat it too, alongside pickles, *dal* and pizza. Within this culinary montage, identity is uncertain and sometimes risky, circulating between insider and outsider, home and abroad, there and back again. In her first interview, Parvati Gowda (43) said of the changing identity of her seventy-eight-year-old mother, Meenakshi: 'Initially she used to like pizza and stuff and [then] there was a stage where she was, "No I want rice". If we go out, she would want rice. She would insist, "Call the waiter and ask him – I want rice". Now she's *back*. Now she doesn't mind eating anything (emphasis added).'

Ageing and Eating

Within this flavoursome landscape, the ageing body represents the gendered embodiment of nostalgia, through the benevolent and kindly mother or grandmother preparing home-cooked meals. Ironically, while this kindly old figure might prepare 'hot' foods – spicy and fried – these cooks are not meant to consume these dishes, instead eating 'cooler', more age appropriate foods. Traditionally in the *vanaprastha* and *sanyas* life stage, an older person's disengagement from everyday life was symbolized in part through increased regulation and austerity of diet. Older people were meant to eat simpler, plainer food and their appetites have been described in terms of frugality and wholesomeness: Cohen's (1998) poorer participants ascribed the weakness of their ageing relatives to the few *rotis* they could feed them; Vatuk's (1990: 75) older people claimed to only want 'two pieces of bread a day' to survive; while Lamb's (2000: 139) village participants spoke disparagingly of a ninety-year-old woman's desire for mangoes, sweets and cottage cheese.

If displaying overt interest in food is seen as age inappropriate, then eating has long been a strategy by which older people transgress their life course. This is best evidenced in the epicurean richness of Indian film and fiction, which features older people eating and demanding age inappropriate foods (Raja 2005). For example, in the film *Pather Panchali* (1955), based on the 1929 novel by Bibhutibhushan Banerjee, the old aunt Indir is first introduced to the audience by her hands, feet and appetite. We see her crouched over her bowl of *dal* and rice, which she mixes and mashes with gusto before enthusiastically devouring it. Her obvious relish and joy for treats like guavas and bananas sits in contrast to the poverty of the household and prompts a rebuke from the young mother of the house, 'You eat the fruit . . . you should know better . . . you think you can do as you please living with us'.

In my sample, in a south Delhi suburb, another *Pather Panchali* was unfolding: the family of ninety-two-year-old Lakshmi Kumari Kochar complained of her constant demands for food, juice and tea. For Lakshmi, these were performative aspects of *sevā* and she claimed food as her right based on her non-working *hāth-pair* because of her dementia and her age. Her hunger fluctuated according to her age – she claimed to be eighteen, fifty and eighty years old on the multiple occasions I met her – and as her age increased, so did her appetite. Also on the increase was her family's concern about managing her weight, mobility and urinary incontinence. They repeatedly tried to control her diet, but to little effect. Lakshmi remained insatiable and intractable, complaining to neighbours and guests that her daughter-in-law did not feed her. Embarrassment and anger were inevitable. By my third visit to the family, they no longer conversed with Lakshmi but commanded her, 'Get up, change your clothes! Come out of the bathroom, stop wasting water!' Lakshmi ignored these instructions and in addition to demands for food, insisted that her hair be dyed black. This caused further rancour. Her sixty-nine-year-old daughter-in-law grumpily remarked, 'In nineties, what need is there for all this image consciousness?'

The real and imaginary stories of Lakshmi and Indir respectively illustrate that eating is a powerful way to continue to hold onto life, unsettle identity, resist the transitions of age and the losses that accompany it. For older people who are no longer the centre of household affairs, eating is pleasurable, vital, therapeutic and symbolic of intergenerational reciprocity and *sevā*. Vandhana Arora (38) highlighted this when she described the epicurean interactions between her mother-in-law, Mrigakshi (74), and her oceanographer father-in-law, A.P. Arora (79): 'She is in the kitchen cooking and he is in the bedroom. From there he is shouting and the best part is he calls her "Darling". Anyway, so from the bedroom, he's calling her, "Darling" and asking, "Is the food ready? Is the food ready?"'

Gender and Discipline

Cooking and eating are ways to give and receive care, organize daily life and retain citizenship within the domestic sphere. These are also gendered divisions of labour as it is women, especially daughters-in-law, who are meant to show *sevā* to their elders through the preparation of food, deference to their husbands by eating after them and love for their children by nurturing them with their own hands and breast milk in infancy (Chaudhary and Bhargava 2006; Lamb 2000).

Much has been written of the changing role of women in urban India, their careers, consumption, increased independence and changing expectations of familial, marital and romantic relationships (see Das 1988; Kakar 1988; Lau 2006; Thapan 2000; Uberoi 1998). Undoubtedly Indian women and men of all ages are negotiating changing gender roles at a time of heightened global flux and socio-cultural and economic interchange with other, often Western, nations. Amid these processes, there is a burgeoning realization that the established 'shifts' that women perform in the West are also impacting on middle-class Indian women's capacity to undertake paid work, housework, childrearing and to manage the health of husbands, children and elders. In a television advertisement for women's Horlicks® (malted milk powder) a young woman is featured planning her day – organize her husband's office party, supervise the housework, handle her colleague's heartbreak, carpool for her children, write to her aunt – until she suddenly realizes: 'Apne se list me, apna naam nahi [that my own name is missing from my list], Women's Horlicks®, because your body needs you too'.

Within this paradigm, bodies become the site of care, the source where love is taken and given. Women's bodies are often the primary source of carework; their arms cook for their elders, their stomachs are hollow when they fast for their husbands and their breasts heavy when babies are to be fed. The power in cooking, feeding and fasting echoes Foucault's (1980) maxim that power is everywhere, exercised by everyone. Women's bodies, like the bodies of men, children and the aged, are written upon and enter into a mechanics of discipline, invested, marked and trained for carework (Foucault and Sheridan 1977). But if the arms, hunger and breasts of women (re)produce disciplinary foods, then the stomachs of men, children and the old must also be disciplined to eat these foods. Yet, as the Horlicks® advertisement suggests, this is not a one-way transfer of strength: women's bodies need replenishment and nourishment in order to provide this labour. A productive, healthy body, rather than a sacrificial one, is emphasized. Thus, the advertisement concludes with the young woman running and doing yoga, being fit and healthy.

Just as the bodily strength of women is appropriated to care and bolster others, so too women are mobilized to supervise the dietary needs of people with dementia. In the majority of families (n=18), women either cooked or oversaw the cooking by others (e.g., domestic servants or younger women). Their days were structured by food routines, which although commonplace amongst many families in India, was not invisible work. Women and their families recognized the importance of cooking and eating. However, it was only when I encountered an anomaly – Shivbaksh Chand – that the complexities involved in daily food preparation became evident. Because of his wife Helen's dementia, eighty-seven-year-old Shivbaksh had become the chief homemaker. He described cooking for Helen as the most important and valuable task he could do:

> *Breakfast*
> I get up at 5 A.M. in the morning. Then I make tea, then I go for a walk to buy the milk, then I make *khichri* for us – I feed her – then I walk again. Then I do the sweeping and the swabbing, then I go and read the paper. Then I make tea and drink another cup.
>
> *Lunch*
> At about 12 P.M. I soak the rice for lunch and start cooking. I start cutting the vegetables, boiling the *dal*, peeling the garlic and putting it and the *masa:la:s* in the mixxie [blender]. I'll make *dal*, I'll make rice or I'll make the *rotis*; I'll eat one *roti* and she'll eat two.
>
> *Tea*
> In the afternoon I rest till 3:30 P.M. then again I drink tea. In the evening again it [cooking] starts. I'll put the milk on to boil in the small cooker, I'll put it on slow so I don't have to keep an eye on it. After it is heated then I set the *dahi* [yoghurt]. I keep some aside for later in the night.
>
> *Dinner*
> Then I sit and talk to her, we eat and drink and I have a little alcohol. Here see this [shows his bottle of whisky]. *Haa*, I drink one peg [every night]. At 10 P.M. we both drink one, one cup of milk and go to sleep. Then get up in the morning, *chalta hai* life [like this life goes on].

Shivbaksh spent his days in a routine of soaking, chopping, kneading, grinding and stirring, procuring milk and setting yoghurt, making *rajma* in winter and *lauki* (bottle gourd) in summer, parsimoniously drinking one peg of whisky every night while Helen freely smoked her *bi:ṛi:s* (unfiltered cigarettes) (see Fig. 5.1).

In cooking and caring, there is power and discipline in producing and consuming food, adhering to routine, monitoring the person with dementia and self-surveillance for managing time and completing daily tasks. Cooking required detailed planning of daily menus to ensure nutritional balance and variation in main meals, snacks and beverages. The seasonal availability and affordability of ingredients affected these plans as did geography. Many families sought to prepare food that invoked their regional homeland or 'native place' – Keralite Radha Menon cooked tomato rice on Tuesdays, Jaspreet Kaur from Punjab rolled hot *parathas* for breakfast and Bengali Shilpi Mukherjee ordered fish for lunch a few times each week.

Alongside the efforts required to plan and procure ingredients and their nutritional and nostalgic capacities to evoke particular regional identities, the freshness and tastiness of food were also disciplinary measures. Dishes

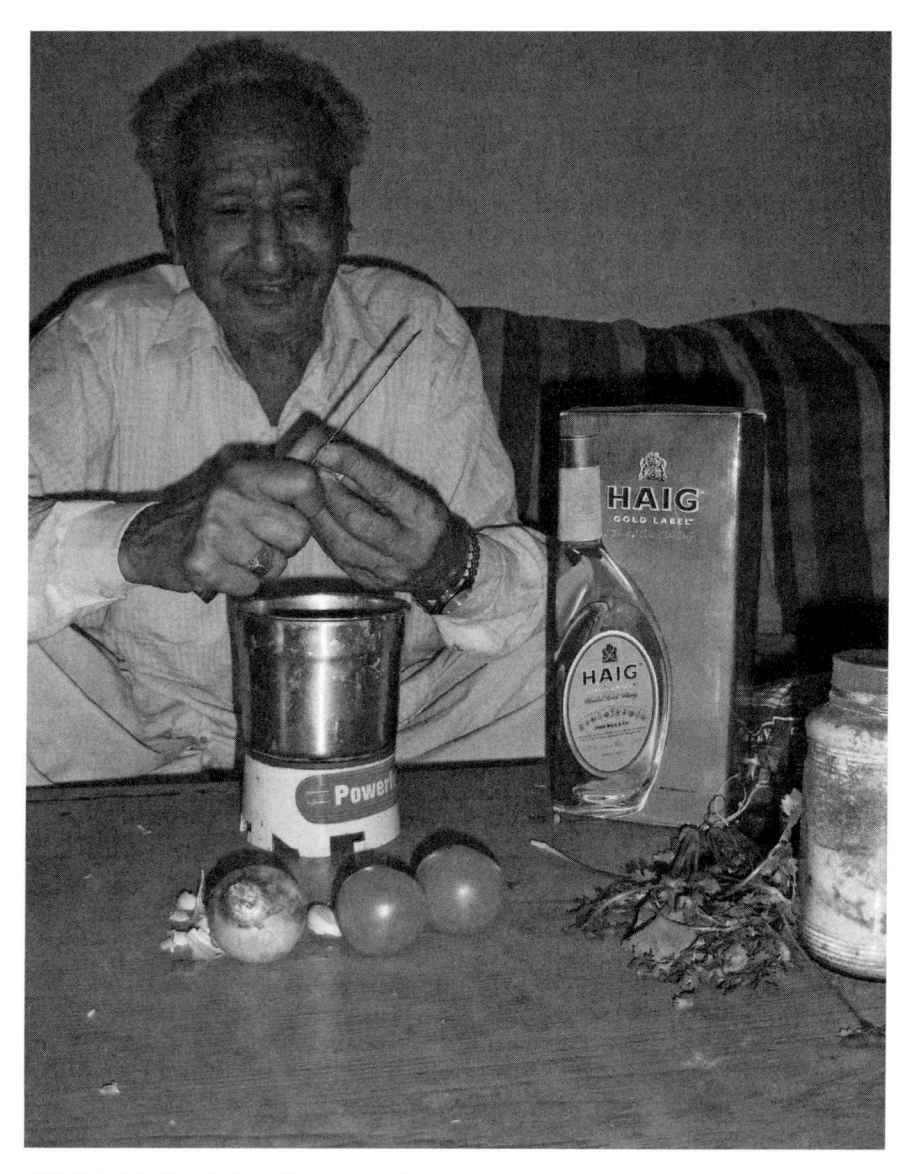

FIGURE 5.1 Shivbaksh Chand cooking

tended to be prepared every day and before each meal, rather than just once a day. The fluffiness of rice, the heat and moisture of *rotis*, the crunchiness of *pakoras*, were all contingent on the immediacy of their preparation and were tied to *sevā*. A caring household was one where there was a daily tri-cyclical performance of preparation, serving and flavour in each meal. These performative aspects not only informed gastropolitics around family dinner tables, but also served as markers of loneliness in social policy. A senior member of India's largest aged care NGO, HelpAge India, explained: 'The grandmother may be given food on a plate in a very disdainful way like you would throw food to the stray dogs. Then you're not giving it with love . . . this leads to isolation and loneliness because a human being is a very social animal and is very perceptive of all this.'

Consequently, pre-packaged or ready-made foods were rarely bought and microwaves were an unusual appliance in family homes. In conjunction, because all the families (except Shivbaksh) had some form of domestic help, these servants would at the very least wash dishes and in other cases help to cook and serve meals. But for most families, cooking and preparing meals consumed their entire day. K.L. Chopra's older daughter-in-law, Rubina, who prepared food every day for K.L. and his wife, was not quite so enthusiastic as her younger sister-in-law, Chintu, about the pleasures of cooking: 'In the morning I give them breakfast, then I send tea, then in the afternoon I give them lunch, then in the evening tea, then the food for dinner and then the milk at night. So in the course of preparing all their food my whole day goes . . . It is a difficult situation'.

Health, Waste and Domestic Citizenship

The importance of food as *sevā* underscores the domestic citizenship that people with dementia experience. As defined by Veena Das and Renu Addlakha, domestic citizenship is:

> A focus on kinship not as the extension of familial relations into community, but as the sphere in which the family has to confront ways of disciplining and containing contagion and stigma [that are] . . . located not in (or only in) individual bodies, but rather as 'off' the body of the individual and within a network of social and kin relationships (2001: 512).

The domestic sphere, argue Das and Addlakha (2001), is constantly at risk of becoming overtly political and needs continuous management by caregivers to maintain the status quo. Scholarship utilizing this concept has linked it to disability. Mehrotra and Vaidya (2008), for example, related domestic citizenship to the discourse of personhood, the physicality of the body and identity politics for individuals and families. Gammeltoft (2008) ascertained that it was a strategy of simultaneous inclusion and exclusion by families towards disabled family members and Dossa (2006) found that it was a way of thinking about how families shuttle between domestic and public spaces in meeting the rights and entitlements of their relatives with a disability.

Specifically with dementia, as the disease progressed, so did the risk of disruption. Relationships changed but people with dementia rarely became invisible in their homes even though they might experience heightened techniques of sequestration through reduced mobility and growing incontinence. Even as their role within the household shifted from elder statesman to managed subject, they still continued to occupy a place and space within household affairs. They were very much citizens in their homes with rights and to whom duties were owed. Through the tacit acknowledgement of their status, families sought to fulfil these obligations. As has already been illustrated, a wide array of services were sought whose quality and variety was contingent on affordability – diet, doctors, diapers, attendants and medicines, each with their own associated objective and subjective costs. For many families, these services eventually coalesced into a disciplinary project of containment and surveillance and further highlighted the fact that people with dementia were at once powerful and powerless in the care dynamic.

As well as being a medium of *sevā* and discipline, food was also imbued with medicinal properties and functioned as a meeting point for biomedicine, traditional and transcendental medicines. Nearly all health practitioners recommended dietary changes to help manage bodily decline. Allopathic doctors suggested fruit, juice and vegetables for digestion; traditional practitioners prescribed coconut water, walnuts and almonds for memory; and transcendental healers offered an assortment of spices, chillies and lime to exorcise djinns and other malevolent forces. Although not typical 'drug foods' such as tobacco, sugar, tea and coffee,[4] nor of equal potency, the fruits, nuts and spices mentioned above were meant to function in a similar capacity as a sedative or stimulant. Just as drug foods have been used to enhance worker productivity and minimize bodily distress within a capitalist economy, so too these foods sought to enhance carers' moral standing and minimize disruptive risks within a care economy. In seeking, procuring and preparing these foods, physical and emotional labours were emphasized within the domestic sphere. But unlike the more definite pills, powders and processes of an *ilāj*, carers did not discuss the effects of these foods on the person with dementia. Rather, as Das and Addlakha (2001) point out, these become management techniques for care and containment, concerned more with fulfilling duties and giving *sevā* to an older citizen within the social relations of the household than with the healing properties of these foods on the bodies of people with dementia. In that sense they are 'off' the body. This link is evidenced in Nandini's description of using drug foods to manage her father's dementia:

One got to know about electrolytes. I, as a routine, used to get the electrolyte test done – so he [doctor] used to laugh and say, 'Now you've understood. Suddenly if he [father] gets into a major aggression, you go and check his electrolytes. You've got the hang of what to do'. So when sodium and these imbalances are there, aggression goes up. Then the homeopathic doctor helped me with the diet. Like what kinds of things you should give . . . things like curd being given in the night helps his sleeping. Even if he does not eat any of his food, make sure a bowl of curd goes in or a *lassi* goes in and a banana.

In managing aggression and sleep through diet, Nandini uses biomedical and traditional medicine techniques and explicitly links diet and managing her father's aggression within a health discourse. Such a strategy was not uncommon within my sample, but it was more in managing incontinence that diet and health were linked. Fifteen families grappled with urinary and faecal incontinence on a daily basis. In twelve families women were the only cleaners. In two families the cleaning was shared between women and men and only in the Chand family did Shivbaksh help Helen to clean herself. With the exception of a few cases, incontinence was not mentioned unless explicitly asked about. However, unlike the families in Lamb's (2000) work, who viewed incontinence as an accepted part of old age and *sevā*, most carers dealing with incontinence found it an emotional rather than physical challenge that left them angry and drained.

Nowhere is the work of containment and emotional management more visible than in the invisible work of cleaning. Dealing with dirt and its associates – urine, faeces, vomit, sweat, pus – is a form of carework rarely discussed, physically and mentally distanced by those who perform such work and highly sequestered from everyday society (Isaksen 2002; Lawton 1998; Lee-Treweek 1997; Peake, Manderson and Potts 1999; Shaji et al. 2003; Twigg 2000). Such dirt threatens the established order, the discreteness of individual bodies, evokes fear of contagion and the sensation of disgust. Intellectually and morally, people are squeamish about such a topic and sensory anthropology may well have found its descriptive limitations for little has been written sensorially about excretion. But such an anthropology must focus on the symbolic and visceral, in all its sensuality and sordidness (Holtzman 2006). The grinding work of care cannot be wholly understood if we are to shirk away from one of its most onerous tasks, nor can one appreciate the dirty depths of love and *sevā* that people perform for those who have forgotten how and where to go to the toilet:

> Touch wood his [husband] potty is not thin. If he gets diarrhoea then it's very difficult, everything becomes filthy. At least if it's normal then it's just his clothes that are dirtied. The smell is there. He's an adult and if you go to

the toilet once every seven to eight days, then it is going to smell. The whole house stinks. What to do? I have to clean it. See I don't know when he's going to do it, so who can I call to clean it? He can go today, tomorrow, now. Day before yesterday he did a little. I saw it and changed him. Then I checked a little later and there was more. So I cleaned it again. Two hours later, I asked him, 'Has your latrine come?' 'No'. But when I checked there was so much. Then I had to scrub and clean everything, put Dettol®, soak it all. I normally have tea and bread in the evening but that evening my throat was – Anyway now it won't come for another three to four days. Last year in January for eight days, he didn't urinate or excrete. The catheter wasn't on then. For eight days there was nothing and he wouldn't even drink water and would scream with pain. Then after the enema he couldn't stop for two days, his system was so blocked. It was terrible, terrible and it was cold. Touch wood this year that didn't happen (*Sita Aggarwal, 63*).

Disgust is the typical sensory response to dealing with human waste and much carework is centred on minimizing disgust by managing dirt. Disgust has had a long, albeit implicit, history in anthropology; Steiner (1956) wrote about taboo and the sociology of danger, Douglas (1966) about dirt as disorder and matter out of place and Miller (1997) has described disgust as sensorial and relational. It is sensorial in that it is located in our bodily responses to disgust – grimacing, spitting and shuddering – and relational because it is other people's dirt, rather than our own, which is viewed as polluted. Isaksen (2002) has argued that disgust is also time sensitive and that as one engages constantly with taboo bodily fluids over time, feelings of disgust cannot be avoided. In adding to the definition and evolution of disgust – as dirt, sensorial, relational, taboo and time bound – disgust is also spatially prescribed and a part of stigma. There are dirty and disgusting spaces in the domestic and public sphere, e.g., toilets and garbage bins, for which techniques of isolation and management have developed to minimize disgust, reinforce stigma and contain contagion.

Tempering feelings of disgust is part of the complex emotional labour that carers perform when cleaning. As Sita described, this work is harrowing and deeply intimate. Only she changed her husband. This was not unusual, for though nearly all families had some level of assistance, in only six cases did the attendant help with toileting. Families strived to avoid 'accidents' whenever possible, but mess was inevitable at one point or another. Then, as Nandini describes, it could take up to three hours to clean the mess:

You're dealing with his emotions, you're also dealing with your own emotions at the time because you're really cut up with yourself, with all that has happened, you're cut up with everybody, you're angry with everybody. Part of your brain is saying, 'Ok, just shut up and deal with this'. So you tell him, 'Lift your leg here, lift your leg this side' and he's not able to because he is in that panic mode. It's not just about cleaning up. It's also about that state of mind that the person gets into, this pressure that has built around it.

In spite of the difficulties associated with changing and cleaning, carers continued to perform this task. There was constant monitoring for bedsores, groin rashes and bacterial infections. When describing daily routines, nearly all the families mentioned massages and exercise, bathing, sponging and regular turning on the bed. These activities, when combined with cooking and feeding, illustrate the complicated daily routine that carers and people with dementia were engaged in, the recognition of rights and the fulfilment of duties. It also highlights that carework has many tempos: the brassiness of diagnostics, prescriptions and OPDs rests alongside the hum of citizenship and *sevā* within the home and in between 'regimes of normalcy and ways of being are fashioned [that] capture both the densities of localities and the rawness of uniqueness' (Biehl 2004: 478).

'I Want Her to Eat'

> Famine?
> Where is famine?
> Sticking charred to the palate of this land
> roasting in the burning sands
> you unfortunate dwellers of villages and hamlets
> of huts and hovels,
> why did you take birth in this infernal land?
> – *Kāl*, Rawat Saraswat (1970, translated into *Famine* by I.K. Sharma)

Eventually people with dementia stop eating. There are many reasons for this – distraction during mealtimes, refusal to eat, neurological difficulty in recognizing food, diminished olfactory sense, inability to open one's mouth, reduced levels of plasma and brain neuropeptide Y and brain neuroepinephrine (that stimulate appetite), depression and acceptance of death (Marcus and Berry 1998). Inability or refusal to eat amongst older people with dementia tends to be viewed as the starting point for discussions about end of life care in the West. Carers are given choices between tube feeding versus no feeding and pain minimization. Some people opt for the latter based on ideas of comfort, quality of life and a 'good' death.

In India, however, the notion that the inability to eat might signal a family decision about time and means of death was incomprehensible. No family within my sample considered such an option. All those whose relatives were in the late to end stages of dementia chose the nasogastric feeding tube. As Shivbaksh stated unequivocally, 'Whether you understand this as *sevā* or as her being with me, being together, *I want her to eat*' (emphasis added).

Starvation and the diminishing appetite leading to it were viewed with grave concern. Although families repeatedly mentioned this to me, I never fully appreciated the import of these anxieties until I received a phone call at 10:30 P.M. on a balmy Saturday night. The caller was Garima Dawar, whom I'd met four months ago in the Cornwall OPD where I had unsuccessfully tried to recruit her into my study, as a carer for her ageing father. Rushed and uninterested at the time, she perfunctorily took my phone number but when I followed up, she questioned her suitability as an interviewee, explaining that her father had Parkinson's disease and that she had no knowledge of Alzheimer's disease or any other dementia. Taking my cue, I thanked her for her time, assumed that was the end of our association and hung up. But with this phone call, Garima, her voice high and stressed, renewed our connection and sought advice. Her father's memory had deteriorated; he was anxious, paranoid and violent, experiencing urinary incontinence, but worst of all, according to her, he refused to eat. Near tears, frustrated and desperate for an answer, she had telephoned every Cornwall doctor she knew – I was the last desperate straw she clutched and the only one who had answered my phone. She was feeding her father *rotis* and oats every few hours, successfully coaxing down only a few mouthfuls. What should she do?

With little advice to dispense and no one to call upon at that hour, I advised her to put a rubber sheet under her father, to try and feed him something nourishing every few hours rather than a full meal and not to argue with him but to let him talk about old memories. I promised to send her the caregiver's booklet in Hindi the following day, told her that someone from ARDSI-DC would contact her and encouraged her to persevere in trying to contact the Cornwall doctors the following morning. More placated by talking than by my advice, she hung up, promising to call back should she need to. But she never did and I spent the night despairing about the futility of anthropology, wondering instead why I did not become a doctor.

This profound distress that families experienced when people with dementia stopped eating requires elucidation, for a shift occurs from the sweetness of nostalgia, the yearning for home cooking or food as 'mother made it' to a more bitter palate shaped historically by deprivation and hunger. Though they are separate words in English, in Hindi, the word *bhu:kh* denotes starvation and hunger. Rejecting food signalled physical and social decline; it denied a critical component of *sevā* and upset domestic routines and markers of citizenship. Six months after my first interview with her, Parvati Gowda's mother stopped eating:

> It's the eating part which is causing a lot of tension. She is not eating enough. I have to make sure that she is eating properly and every few hours because if I forget, she's not going to tell me she is hungry. Before, every few hours she used to say, 'I am hungry'. But now I have to really monitor.

Shafia, whose husband Omar was on a nasogastric tube when I met them, described how she began to handfeed Omar:

> Once he stopped speaking, when he would eat, sometimes it would go in his mouth and sometimes it would fall down, even dry *rotis*. We put a napkin on him and the food on a tray but he still could not eat it, he dropped it. Slowly we realized that his stomach would never be full, he would become *kāmzor* [weak].

The visible bodily process of hunger – growling stomach, thinness, *kāmzori* – occupies a powerful place within the Indian social imagination. Two reasons explain this preoccupation: (1) a shared history and memories of famine and the continued lived reality of hunger and malnutrition; and (2) the 'right to food' within Hinduism.

In India, famines, hunger and starvation have had a long history,[5] which in part has influenced the development of such a complex structure around food and eating. As Khare points out, a myth of 'immanent abundance' has needed to be perpetuated in order to dissipate 'the actual dimensions of collective scarcity' (1976: 169).

India's last substantial famine was the Great Bengal Famine in 1943, estimated to have resulted in the deaths of between 1.5 and 3 million people (Sen 1981). With Independence, investment and technological innovation in the agricultural sector, famines have declined with the introduction of grain hybrids, higher yields and greater crop resilience to drought and floods. Yet hunger has not disappeared. We must distinguish between famine and starvation, for starvation still occurs within a time of plenty. 'Starvation', writes Amartya Sen, implies 'poverty, since the absolute dispossession that characterizes starvation is more than sufficient to be diagnosed as poverty, no matter what story emerges from the view of *relative* deprivation' (1981: 39). In collaborations with Jean Drèze, Sen (1989, 1990, 1995) has further demonstrated that starvation is more a question of affordability and access to food than shortages in supply.

Endemic hunger, persistent malnutrition and starvation continue to affect India's populations; the root causes are poverty, corruption, high food prices and ineffectual storage and distribution mechanisms (Currie 2000; Mooij 1999; Radhakrishna and Subbarao 1997). Currently nearly half of all Indian children under three are malnourished and more than half of all Indian women are anaemic; these figures exceed those reported in sub-Saharan Africa (UNICEF 2009). Localized famines continue in India, driven by drought, preference for cash over food crops and poverty. Famines are now linked to debt and the disturbing rate of farmer suicides. Many farmers, unable to repay loans for seeds and pesticides and unable to feed their families, kill themselves by ingesting pesticides, drowning or hanging. From 1997 to 2008, 199,132 farmers killed themselves, a trend mainly concentrated in four states (Maharashtra, Andhra Pradesh, Karnataka and Madhya Pradesh) and showing signs of increasing rather than abating (Sainath 20072013).

But while so much of the country goes hungry, Hindu philosophy stresses that '*Bhojan* (eating and giving food to others to eat) is one of the most important subjects treated in the *Dharmasastra* works' (Kane 1930, 1962: 757). Khare's (1998) analysis of Hindu philosophy indicates that four interrelated factors influence the politics around hunger and eating: (1) *Apadharma*, self-preservation in order to fulfil one's duties to others in times of normality and distress; (2) *Palana-posana* or the need to nurture and protect dependents and the needy; (3) *Yogaksema*, faith in rulers and the divine to protect and provide for the marginalized; and (4) *Annabrahma* (food is God), the notion that to feed others is to feed God. Feeding others, especially the poor, is important in Hinduism, Islam, Sikhism and Christianity. Makeshift tents affiliated with local charities and religious centres dispensing hot meals for free are commonplace in Delhi's landscape.

Amongst the families in my study, feeding those less fortunate was a way of fulfilling one's *dharma*; to celebrate Karamjit's seventy-fifth birthday, he and Nina, accompanied by twenty-two extended family members, decided to feed other people. Nina recounted:

> He was the man of honour and you should have seen him, he was lapping it up, the attention, he was having wine! My God you should have just seen how he was lapping it up, the importance given to him! He loved it, oh my God! You see he's never ever hurt anybody, never ever called anyone names, he's never been nasty, so people have a lot of love for him. All his family – we went to Mathura for his birthday and we fed 6,000 people. He was feeding them – 6,000 people!

Given the centrality of eating and feeding within India politically, economically and philosophically, starvation therefore represents profound unease and unhappiness in the social imagination. Poverty, hunger and starvation are lived realities on India's streets for *all* its citizens. It affects those who are deprived and marginalized in terms of life expectancy, health status, economic opportunity and lived inequalities. Its impact is more symbolic on those with full bellies, for confronting the hungry poor on a daily basis also represents the greatest failure of more powerful people and government to sufficiently fulfil their duties to India's dispossessed. Anxieties surrounding starvation among those living with Alzheimer's are framed against these backdrops and represent a failure outside and inside the home, an inadequacy of middle-class families, not only in effectively responding to the needs of public citizens, but also to their immediate domestic citizens.

Sweetness and Play

Appadurai (1981) has noted that gastropolitics in India is akin to Geertz's description of cockfighting amongst the Balinese – it is a state of deep play involving the moral and medical taxonomy of food with considerable stakes. Because feeding and eating reveal so much about age, identity, gender, discipline, power, hunger, domesticity and citizenship, the risks are so high as to be almost impossible for families to successfully negotiate. Indeed, all the families experienced censorship and failure at one point or another, in nearly all aspects of procurement, preparation and consumption of food. Jaspreet intercepted Harinder eating soap, Savitri hid bananas and oranges from her father-in-law lest he eat them whole before she peeled them and Chintu found her mother-in-law eating stale *rotis* in the kitchen. Success was a delicate dance on shaky ground and there was much at stake. When done 'right', the rewards of feeding made it the most pleasurable aspect of caring for families and nearly all the carers I asked said feeding was the activity they enjoyed the most.

Sweetness and the pleasure of feeding and eating were explicitly linked by seven families who talked about the happiness they derived from feeding and eating sweets. The preference for sugary products among people living with Alzheimer's disease has been noted, but little has been written on the relationality and fun of sugar in such a dynamic. Sugar was a 'treat', a small deviation from the heavy disciplines of health management that families could indulge their loved ones in. Scattered amidst the scripts of diet and care, sugar was a fine, crystallized pleasure. Josie gave Su chocolate, describing it as 'little luxuries', Savitri gave her father-in-law sweets so that he would say '*achchhe se thē* (it was good)', one of only two phrases left in his vocabulary and Suneeta put sugar in her father's *dal* so that he would find it tastier. Eating sweets together was an act that spouses especially enjoyed. Nina said, 'Yesterday we were having ice-cream and I said,

"You've had your fruit, will you have some ice-cream?" and he said, "Oh yes!"'

There is a close link between food and sex, especially in the subcontinent. Sudhir Kakar reminds us 'That in the Indian consciousness, the symbolism of food is more closely or manifestly connected to sexuality than it is in the West' (1990: 78). Eating and sexual enjoyments have the same etymologic root in Sanskrit, *bhuj*, and perform the same task in prescribing and maintaining social order. A growing body of literature is exploring the connection between food and sex in the Asian theatre.[6] However, in my analysis, this connection can at best be inferred in the intimacy and pleasure of feeding, for no carer explicitly linked food and sex and I lacked the courage to ask about this delicate subject. Moreover, as many interviews were frequently interrupted and took place with various family members concurrently participating, the subject could not easily be broached.

Nevertheless, for spouses, eating sweets together was pleasurable and romantic. In his slow methodical voice, Tandon initially described his wife, Sheila's, routine to me – a regimen of healthy diet, medication, exercise and personal hygiene. He and the attendant shared the carework, but at around 8 P.M. every night, once Sheila was put to bed, the attendant departed and he was alone. Lying in the twin bed next to his wife, he would put on the TV, hoping that Sheila would hear something to make her laugh so that she would smile as she drifted into sleep. Eventually he too would sleep but hoped to be awakened at around 3 A.M. by Sheila's laughs. This was the time when she was most responsive and talkative; he would sit, talk and feed Sheila her favourite sweet – ice-cream. Tandon's mouth crinkles and smiles at this memory, this is the best part of his day:

> Sitting with her and talking to her. Uplifting her spirits. Feeding her gives me a lot of [happiness]. It is my heart's desire to feed her, to feed her from my heart, in peace, with love, to give her food. These are my most favourite activities. She knows that I am feeding her from my hands. She responds to me, I can see her reaction, talk to her.

Feeding and eating are sites of deep play also because they represent the flavours of deep love. In the oceanographer asking his darling 'what's for lunch?', Josie feeding Su chocolate, Shivbaksh's all-consuming cooking for Helen, the Bhagat's dinner table desserts and Tandon's secret interludes in the wee hours of the morning, love in all its zest and sweetness is visible. The tongue and the taste buds become erogenous zones because of memory not sex. Tasting, feeding and eating are ways in which marriages that are irrevocably changing are held onto. They are also ways in which husbands and wives can transgress the roles of 'carer' and 'person with dementia' and claim the intimacy of giving and receiving pleasure from each other. Sensory anthropology is at its richest here for the sweetness of sugar is experienced bodily and symbolically. Husbands and wives smile, talk and make sounds (like 'mmm') to each other, to connote pleasure with food and each other's company. Symbolically sweetness also temporarily alleviates the bitterness of memory and loss of function. In deep play, sugar sits at the unfathomable bottom, in a hard to reach place, neither mired in health nor citizenship, promising sweetness and love. Little wonder that food is so critical to the care relationship.

Conclusion

On assembling the ingredients, defining their properties, mixing and separating, we see that when combined, feeding and eating are part of a contradictory feast. Food is sensory, rooted in the body but also off the body, the site of discipline yet transgression, power and also love. Food, in India, is not merely sustenance but the material representation of identity in age and gender as well as a currency of personhood in social exchanges. Cooking, feeding and eating are acts of dominance and subservience, markers of *sevā* and care, which appropriate not just bellies but also breasts, hands and voice. Carers can engage in techniques of management and surveillance of the self and people with dementia.

Starvation and hunger frame the backdrop of this gustatory experience, bringing famine, death and poverty to the table, reminding the feasters that inequities linger more acutely in other physical and social bodies and that eating is as much a political act as it is a pleasurable one. Feeding and eating then, are not just acts necessary for sustenance. Rather, in the subcontinent, food and the appetite are central aspects of care.

Notes

1. Fried unleavened bread made from wholemeal flour and stuffed with cauliflower.
2. *Pao-bha:ji* is a Maharashtrian snack that comprises a *pao* or bread and *bha:ji*, typically a potato based curry. *Gula:b jammuns* are deep fried balls of cottage cheese (or other milk solids) soaked and served in a rose infused sugar syrup.
3. *Rajma-cha:val* is a popular north Indian meal of red kidney beans cooked with spices and served with white rice.
4. See Bradburd and Jankowial (2003), Mintz (1996), Nichter and Thompson (2006) and Stromberg, Nichter and Nichter (2007).
5. Bhatia (1967) estimates that there were fourteen famines in India from the eleventh to seventeenth centuries that killed millions of people (exact numbers are not

available). In the latter half of the nineteenth century, there were about twenty-five major famines believed to have killed between 30 and 40 million people.
6. See, for example, Farquhar's (2002) work in China, Liechty's (2005) in Kathmandu and Alter's (2000) in India.

6. STIGMA AND LONELINESS IN CARE

Indian society doesn't put a stigma on Alzheimer's disease or dementia; it is a part of the ageing process and can happen to anybody. So not much of stigma, just the burden of caring, the load of caring (*Dr Bose, Sarkari Geriatrician*).

Of course there is a lot of stigma. A lot of times we are told, 'Don't come through the front door; come through the rear door because the neighbours will see that there is this kind of patient at home'. So we tell them, 'This is nothing to be ashamed of. Tell your neighbours and your friends that there is a patient like this who has lost his memory' (*P.K. Singh, Volunteer, ARDSI-DC*).

What Alzheimer's disease is, people don't know. How it happens, what age it happens in, people don't know. Often I'm asked what work I do. I never say I work with Alzheimer's patients, I say that I care for mental patients, I handle them (*Sandra Anu, Attendant*).

Sometimes I get tired, 'What a life I have got *yaar*' (*Suneeta Sadhwani, Carer*).

THERE IS CONFUSION ABOUT WHETHER people living with dementia and their families experience stigma. Families and doctors often said that there was no stigma against dementia, while ARDSI would insist that stigma affected relationships in the home and families' relations with the world at large. Although it might be argued that ARDSI had a vested interest in claiming stigma existed – to garner more funds to raise awareness of their organization – this does not present the complete picture. Many within ARDSI worried about the existence of stigma and these anxieties reflect the complex picture that emerges when stigma is examined in India. In my field notes I often noted the contradiction of how carers reported high levels of social support from their communities, while simultaneously describing lonely lives. Many carers were refused offers of marriage for their children and they and the person with dementia were increasingly distanced from the wider community. Equally, people complained of being neglected and alone even as a steady stream of visitors flowed in and out of their home. Shivbaksh Chand said he was alone but made daily visits to the local dispensary across his street to chat with his peers, entertained visitors and tolerated anthropologists in his home. Suneeta Sadhwani said her neighbours were 'very helpful', but in her daily routine cared for her father largely unaided.

The apparent inconsistencies in these stories are largely due to the contrariness of the disease itself. Dementia sits in the juncture between ageing and mental illness and its symptoms may lend themselves to either category. While stubbornness and anger in one's *buddhāpan*, or old age, may have been accepted with ageing, behaviour disruption, violence and disinhibition were more readily interpreted as signs of madness/mental illness and could become grounds for institutionalization. Categories such as 'ageing' and 'madness' constantly risked collapsing in on each other, separated only by the efforts of families and the NGO. 'It is important not to label people with Alzheimer's as mad; they are *ya:dda:sht ke mari:z* [the memory patients]', said P.K. Singh, an ARDSI volunteer, to the residents of a Delhi old age home.

The stigma experienced by families depended on how others perceived them and where they positioned themselves on the scale between ageing and madness. I describe these performative acts of positioning and illustrate how stigma is internalized and deeply felt, externally visible and publicly executed. I do this through an analysis of three local worlds and their moral stakes: individual relations, social processes and institutional practices. I explore how families exercise agency and choice in their responses and resistance to stigma as well as how families and people with dementia stigmatized others (and each other) for perceived 'defects' or marks. In mapping this social geography of stigma it will be shown that stigma is a space in which structure and agency rub against each other in contradictory and uncomfortable ways.

Defining Stigma

Erving Goffman (1959, 1990), in his seminal work, defined stigma as a deeply discrediting attribute located not so much in an individual as within social relationships. A person is assigned a negative characteristic – physical abnormality, failure of character, tribal stigma (such as race, religion, nationality) – that a larger social group then uses as the basis to discredit and exclude them. Such an interpretation of stigma has been widely applied across disciplines and topic areas. Jones (1984) added to this definition by describing attributes that 'marked' people as deviant within particular social contexts and Crocker and colleagues (1998) extended it to show that stigma was socially constructed and that an individual's social identity was devalued in particular societies in specific ways.

These definitions of stigma have been criticized for centring too much on individual attributes and characteristics, without attending to the structural factors that exclude and discriminate (Parker and Aggleton 2003). Albeit closely related, stigma and discrimination are not the same. The former is a deeply discrediting attribute, while the latter is a set of actions by which the stigmatized individual's life opportunities are reduced (Reidpath, Brijnath and Chan 2005). Discrimination and stigma tend to flow along established rivulets of power and inequality and institutions tend to discriminate against people not only on the basis of their stigmatized attributes but also by class, gender and race (Parker and Aggleton 2003). Therefore, any discussion of stigma also needs to examine institutional discriminations to understand the mechanisms of social control and its deleterious effects on the lives of people who are stigmatized.

Link and Phelan (2001) have incorporated these criticisms, arguing that stigma is a process comprising five interrelated stages: (1) initially people distinguish themselves from each other through labels (e.g., race, gender, sexual preference); (2) a negative stereotype is then assigned to particular labels; (3) those who are labelled are then separated from 'us'; (4) they are viewed as less than 'us' and experience a loss of status; and (5) they are likely to be marginalized through the institutional power of the state.

Link and Phelan's work has resonated with Arthur Kleinman's writing on social suffering, local worlds and moral exigencies. Kleinman (1991, 1999, 2006) delves into how social experiences are lived in particular local worlds, identifying the stakes, strategies and pragmatic responses of people to threats and dangers. To be stigmatized, he argues, is to experience social suffering – a term he, Lock and Das (1997: ix) describe as the 'assemblage of human problems that have their origins and consequences in the devastating injuries that social force can inflict on human experience'. Violence and trauma constitute part of the suffering that people and societies may inflict on each other to preserve an established order. Also emphasized is the role of state apparatus in creating suffering, stigma and social death. Kleinman's work in China shows that social death can mean the disintegration of the existence, value and perpetuity of the individual and the family (Lee et al. 2006; Yang and Kleinman 2008).

Recent collaborations between Link, Phelan, Kleinman and their colleagues (2007) have centred on amalgamating moral experience into stigma theory. 'Moral experience', they write, 'refers to that register of everyday life and practical engagement that defines what matters most for ordinary men and women' (Yang et al. 2007: 1528). Further, they argue, stigma threatens what matters most, occurs in an inter-subjective space between people and also in individual bodies whether consciously acknowledged or not. In other words, it necessitates multiple methods and perspectives in order to fully capture its complexity in theory, social attitudes and praxis.

To this definition of stigma, I would also add that moral experiences vary according to their local worlds, which transpire in particular socio-geographical spaces. What is at stake in the clinic is not the same as what is chanced in marriage negotiations, nor what is experienced within a household when bodily disintegrations are perceived as polluting. In each setting, physical and social boundaries change, as do techniques of avoidance and boundary maintenance (Douglas 1966). Thus, different forms and gradations of stigma play out, executed in words and in acts, which mobilize bodies differently in public and private spaces. To understand these mobilizations, their significance and the use of space, a deliberately under deterministic language is necessary. Stigma may be blatant in institutions and some human relations but can also be subtle, residing in understated gestures, which, when compiled, show a deep, long-term, grievous hurt. Similarly, acts of exclusion and insult, which can be seen as stigma, may have their genesis in other paradigms. In the clinic, when families are asked if their older relative has psychosis, in front of med reps and other patients, it may be because the patient is seen to be mad. But it can also be explained through a range of other factors such as an authoritarian doctor-patient relationship, high patient demand and/or the pressure to multitask in order to manage heavy workloads. Similarly, prescriptions for antipsychotics may be offered not because the person has psychosis, but because a doctor receives kickbacks from pharmaceutical companies (see chapter 4). Indeed, things are never what they seem when praxis is contextualized by space; a point that Deleuze articulates well: 'Something strange happens, something that blurs the image, marks it with an essential uncertainty, keeps the form from "taking", but also undoes the subject, sets it adrift and abolishes any paternal function. It is only here that things begin to get interesting' (1998: 77).

Preserving the Normal

Many families were engaged in a project to preserve the normal and avoid the indignities of stigma. Through the acts of daily living, such as bathing, dressing and feeding, they strived to maintain identity and contain disruption. In the early days of my fieldwork, people with dementia were presented to me in particular ways: K.P. Aggarwal was dressed in an immaculate white *kurta:* when I first met him, Mrs Hamdari had on her pearl earrings and K.L. Chopra took out silk suits for his wife, Meera, to wear on the day of my first visit to their home. The beautification was done just prior to my arrival. Often people's hair was still damp but neatly combed, there was a fresh smell of soap, white powder was dusted on their necks and there were no wrinkles in their clothes. People who could no longer walk were propped up in bed; those who were still mobile would be brought in for the duration of the interview or early on for me 'to see' them and comment upon their care. Though disconcerting, this was a strategy whereby families maintained a veneer of normalcy towards strangers. In my second interview with Bhageshwari, she brought her mother, Tara, into the room and spent fifteen minutes attempting to get Tara to recall her (Bhageshwari's) name. Finally Tara remembered.

> My name starts with 'B'. I know you'll tell me. 'B'
> Bhageshwari's your name
> See, you know my name. I know you can't forget me. You can't forget my name
> If that's your name
> [To BB] *See?* Touchwood that way she's very cheerful (emphasis added)

Families worked hard to steer their relatives away from the label of madness through invoking the sensory measurement of sight. People with dementia were not mad, they were normal, and if one sat down and engaged with them, one could *see* this. Asking people to engage with people with dementia to see how normal they were was a technique by which those who might stigmatize could verify through their own experiences how far removed people with dementia were from madness. Families used the sight metaphor as a measure of this engagement – they used words like '*dekhnā:*' in Hindi, 'see' and 'face-to-face' in English. Seeing became a tactic through which to subvert the gaze that would label madness. Radha Menon, who struggled with her husband's violence and fluctuating moods, explained: '*Pa:gaal* means to walk around the street without clothes. But he doesn't take off his clothes. *You've seen?* He talks in a good way. Just his behaviour we have to manage a little. I have to have patience, to talk properly, to talk in a peaceful manner' [emphasis added].

Downplaying Alzheimer's and emphasizing the normal was a tactic to anchor disruption in the 'normal' difficulties of ageing and mitigate against the stigma of madness. It was not that carers were in denial; by this point they had accepted the disease. This was mostly clearly reflected in their use of language. In Hindi, chronic diseases are generally referred to in the present tense and language plays a key role in how the sick role comes to colonize the entire identity of the person. Mental *hai*, sugar *hai*, heart *hai* (is mental, is diabetic, is a heart problem) was how illnesses were usually ascribed by other people onto the sick person. There was little use of progression or tense – it was not *ho gaya:* (it has happened) but *hai* (it is). The use of the present tense highlights the ontological shifts that occur in perception. People become indivisible from their illness and their former identities divorced from their present states. 'Normal' is a distant shore on which identity is left stranded and people are now seen as demented, diabetic and faulty hearts. Language becomes one way by which signs of illness become scripted onto and embodied within people. Language functions as a social symbol, providing information and cues about how sick people should be read and perceived within society (Goffman 1963, 1986).

Interestingly, the word 'problem' was hardly ever used in the constitution of this new sick role. Rather, 'problem' referred to things that could be fixed, applied to temporal conditions and specific body parts and processes such as leg pain, toothaches and headaches. Carers often described their own health concerns as 'problems' or applied the term to conditions where an *ilāj* could be sought to redress the problem.

However, in trying to preserve normality, families did not seek to bleach out the identity of the person with dementia just as in 'seeing' madness outsiders did not immediately seek to ostracize people with dementia. While the 'gaze' as an exercise in power, discipline and conformity was brought to bear on the person with dementia, for carers, the gaze was also an entry point into performance and pleasure (Foucault and Sheridan 1977; Goffman 1961). Disruptions were concealed in order to produce finished, polished images not just to preserve the image of the normal, but also because there was pleasure to be gained from beautification (Goffman 1959: 52–53). This 'discipline of normalization' was productive, transformative and creative, rather than repressive (Foucault 1975, 2003: 52). Families wanted their loved ones to look fresh and smart to outsiders, they enjoyed combing hair, dabbing powder and selecting silk clothes. They spent money on clothes, cosmetics and soaps, cleaned mess, hid the 'dirty work' that went into producing this image and sacrificed their own body to dirt and disorder. To view these solely as acts of conformity disregards the love in these acts of *sevā*. For Kumud Kaul, who cared for her mother, Mrs Hamdari, love was a key factor in her striving for normalcy: 'So just before she is wearing her clothes I tell the girl, "Keep *nani's* clothes ready and nice," and so it's ironed and she'll get dressed. That is what I love'.

Normality and Danger

But asking outsiders to see normality was a risky approach. Ironically, the stakes hinged on the person with dementia behaving *too* normal. Claims of illness rested on the abnormality of the engagement and some anomaly had to be produced to substantiate such an assertion. To be *seen* to be normal was not to be normal. As time went by and my relationships with families deepened, certain bodily enactments of normality dropped off and I began to see signs of disruption: urine bags, catheters, sweat, faded clothes and mussed hair.

People with dementia were expected to be forgetful, a little vague and eccentric. When they were not, carers could sometimes grow defensive. When I engaged with Radha's husband, Rajesh, we talked about his desire to return to Kerala, his wish to work, what he had eaten for lunch, his background and political leanings. In other words, Rajesh spoke normally. However, Radha found this conversation deeply troubling. She interpreted it as evidence for me to question the authenticity of her claims about Rajesh's dementia and said defensively:

> [Angry voice] Sometimes people don't understand. What do they think – that I am going to speak lies about my husband and say he isn't well? Sir sometimes speaks nicely. That's why nobody believes me. Nobody can believe that.
> *Who says this?*
> Some of the friends who come to visit. They don't believe me. I tell them, 'Am I mad to say such things about my *a:dmī:* (husband)?'

When ears were tuned to hear senility and illness and instead heard the articulate speech of the elder, the carer's character came into question. The questions of integrity and madness were passed onto the carer and they would have to defend themselves against the sudden scrutiny. For example, Radha's angry testimony – 'Am I mad to say such things about my *a:dmī:* ?' – illustrates that people did view her askance because Rajesh did not always behave unusually. Importantly, this judgement applied only in the early stages of the illness; later, as diminished mobility, incontinence and lost speech became more visible, such questions were no longer relevant. But in the interim, which could be as long as ten years, families walked a tightrope between normal/ill and ageing/madness. They sought to anchor the person with dementia's identity in the normal ageing body rather than in the *pa:gaal's* body, but staked their own claims to care in illness and ageing.

Preserving too much normality was a hazard that carers faced not just with outsiders but also with family members. Some family members were not entirely convinced about the dementia, despite diagnosis and medication, but were hesitant about airing their doubts. In the Chopra family, for example, a familial narrative of diagnosis and care was initially presented to me – the proverbial story of strangeness, crisis, diagnosis, acceptance, *sevā*, care and familial cohesion. In my first interview with K.L. Chopra, his wife Meera, their two daughters-in-law and a distant older aunt were co-contributors to this unified tale. Even the local postman arrived midway to nod sagely as Chopra enthusiastically spoke about his 'settled' (i.e. married and gainfully employed) children who did so much *sevā* for him and Meera. Three months later, time and the May sun had wilted nearly everyone's research fervour and only Chopra and his elder daughter-in-law, Rubina, were present for our interview. The tale of the good family remained consistent – all the adult children were settled and performed the appropriate amount of *sevā*. However, when I went upstairs to Rubina's flat for lunch, I found myself briefly alone with her. She hurriedly spoke:

> There is nothing wrong with mummy. She knows everything – who's coming, who's going, what is hers, where it is, who has what – she knows everything. *Baas* [finished] it is just that daddy gives her so many medicines that she has become like this. And her younger son is not good. *See*, you sat there for one hour and he came in once but he never sat down or offered you a cup of tea. He won't sit and talk. And his wife is busy in her job all the time (emphasis added).

In Rubina's secret narrative, Meera was not 'mental', i.e., she had neither dementia nor mental illness. Rather, her problems were attributed to medication and modernity. Too many drugs, a working daughter-in-law and a bad son; Cohen's (1998) work echoes as the good family suddenly reveals its bad side. All one had to do, according to Rubina, was to *see* it. Meera's familiarity with her surroundings and her son's inhospitality were to be seen as signs of a bad family and not of mental deviance.

Other families had similar doubters. Sita Aggarwal's son showed me twenty years of his father's medical history, with multiple confirmed diagnoses of Alzheimer's disease, but still quietly questioned his father's dementia. Shivbaksh thought that eighty-two-year-old Helen's problems could be caused by dementia, but also attributed them to hormones and menopause. After Su died, Josie wondered whether he had Alzheimer's disease or a vitamin deficiency. Within these families, Cohen's (1998) 'bad' families resonated; there were squabbles and tensions with extended relatives and immediate kin. Running alongside was the undercurrent of hope, the desire for the dementia diagnosis to be replaced by some other condition for which there was hope for a cure. Even in cases where the person with dementia had died, carers still sought an alternative etiology so that they could offer hope to other families.

Thus sight and seeing functioned as a contrary tactic – a way of acknowledging normality, but also sickness and madness. In giving outsiders the opportunity to see for themselves families risked much and therefore sought to overlay their own perceptions of sight and family politics on the external gaze. As Radha Menon put it, 'You have to care for him, bring him tea, tell him, "Drink it, eat your food" . . . you just have to give him everything. [But] there are no problems – you can *see* it, can't you?'

Internal and External Stigma

If the project of preserving the normal was about avoiding the stigma of madness it eventually failed because as the disease progressed, performing normality became increasingly difficult and sequestration was commonplace. This was a two-way process where families and carers endured, but also imposed exile on themselves and their interactions with their moral worlds. Stigma became internally and externally enforced, linked to space, bodily function and fear of social censorship.

In the Tandon household isolation stemmed from diminished function. Tandon and Sheila led cloistered lives, reinforced by the geography of their household. They lived on the first floor in a corner plot, up a winding staircase, behind high concrete walls. All their doors and windows had grills. Unless they permitted entry through an imposing black gate, which was locked from the inside, it was physically impossible to get to them. As Sheila's dementia progressed, her world shrank to her bathroom and bedroom. She spent her days being lifted from her bed to her wheelchair and back again. Tandon's life had also shrunk as he grew increasingly preoccupied with the minutiae of his wife's body. He said repeatedly that he was alone. Although they had once enjoyed good relations in their local community, attending marriages and social functions, few friends and neighbours now came to visit. Tandon was philosophical: 'They feel sympathetic. They know me for the last ten years and she was in the good books of the colony. Initially they used to come and inquire about her but now they have stopped because she can't respond to them. So how can they even begin to talk to her?'

In Tandon's world, stigma was not so much a damaging marker as a social distance. The layout of the house, Sheila's lack of responsiveness and Tandon's focus on her all made them difficult to access. They and their neighbours grew increasingly apathetic and disengaged from each other. Tandon himself admitted, 'You will go to people's homes who will respond to you; why will you go where no one will respond to you?' In contrast, the Khan family actively sought to withdraw Omar from their community. They feared that as illness undid him, his reputation as a respected and well-known figure would be spoilt. Shafia explained this failed attempt:

> We didn't like him going out because we didn't want outsiders to mock him. We thought it was better that people did not know of his illness but he would go out. The children would catch him and bring him home, 'Aunty he was here, aunty he was there'. Everyone soon came to know that he was sick, that he had some problem. He was always wandering out without any shoes.

In public spaces, the Tandons and the Khans used a set of defensive and protective practices (Goffman 1959) to maintain the image of the person with dementia and the image of the family. By curtailing Omar's movement, the Khan family sought to preserve a virtual identity of who he was versus the social reality of who he had become. Tandon, through his social and spatial disengagement from his neighbours, sought a similar end. These were not attempts to 'hide' the truth; Omar's wanderings and Sheila's decline were freely known in their communities and had long disrupted the veneer of normalcy. Instead, these were a kind of 'strategic' secret (Goffman 1959), a way of disguising the depths of change and disorder within the household and of obfuscating the capacities of particular family members. Information was held back because of its potential to stigmatize and discredit the household. But in attempting to manage a family image and individuals' identities, families found themselves increasingly isolated through their own internalized stigmas.

To understand the anxiety driving these practices, it is necessary to examine the stakes associated with 'seeing'. In the Khan's case, Omar's physical degeneration was also the decline of the family's social status. This affected their material and social capital. Omar's dementia and his loss of earning capacity put increasing pressure on the family budget and the Khans grew poorer and less able to draw on prior relationships to bolster their income. Former influential friends no longer visited nor provided money; Shafia had approached an old contact for aid and in turn received Rs 1,000 per month for a year. Her son worked as a low-level manager in a telemarketing firm, her older daughters had married and moved elsewhere and her youngest daughters had yet to be settled. Their precarious finances had led to Shafia opening a tailoring shop beneath her flat to bring in extra income. These monetary woes, coupled with Omar's illness, affected the Khan family's capacity to broker marriages with more affluent families and to make the necessary 'gifts' for these successful negotiations. Their income was not enough to overcome the stigma of dementia, here associated with symptoms such as wandering and wearing no shoes.

Those seen to be caring for an ageing, as opposed to sick, family member garnered significant social support. Suneeta Sadhwani (41), the sole carer for her father, Hari Prasad (74), tearfully described how 'nice' people were in her neighbourhood. She related how people assisted her when Hari wandered away for the first time:

> Once when I didn't know that he [father] was forgetting the way, we were coming home and I realized I had forgotten to buy a *dal*. So I said to him, 'Papa, I've forgotten to buy that *dal*, can you please go and pick it up? In the meantime, I'll carry on home'. He went there to the shop, he got the *dal*, but he was so late getting home. An hour had passed and I said to myself, 'It doesn't take an hour to buy *dal*, the market is in front'. I called up our ration *wallah's* shop and I said, 'Uncle, this is what's happened . . . Papa hasn't come home yet. What the *chakkar* (confusion) is I don't understand'. He said, '*Beta* you don't worry, I'll send my assistant out on the scooter to look for him'. I also went downstairs to search and there was his assistant coming on his scooter . . . Now the lane you came down, on the opposite side, someone had left him there. Maybe it's because of God that I get so much cooperation, I don't know, but people are very nice.

Suneeta's ability to gain sympathy and kindness from her community was based on a combination of neighbourhood density, time and Hari's symptoms. They had lived in their west Delhi colony for many decades and were well-known. Suneeta had taught in the local school and still gave private tuition to supplement their income. Their second-floor flat was small and in the middle of the block in a densely packed suburb. Buildings were squashed together and the inside roads were narrow and apartments sprang up on either side. As the Sadhwanis did not have a car, public transport was their only option; the main road, from where buses, auto-rickshaws and trains were available, was a three-minute walk away. To get to public transport, the local market, banks and the post office, one had to walk through the inner lanes of the colony, visible to neighbours from their windows and verandas. Because their income was low and they could not afford to hire a full-time servant to run their errands, Suneeta and Hari walked to as many places as they could. They were a common sight and their comings and goings were readily noticed.

Hari was a quiet, still man who rarely left his home on his own. He got lost easily and, aware of his forgetfulness, he relied heavily on Suneeta to mediate his relations with the outside world. In public, he was neither aggressive nor repetitive and had never been violent. He moved softly and hardly spoke; his communication techniques were restricted to folding his hands and saying *Namaste* or shaking hands. As he was able to fulfil these decorum cues and was not publicly disruptive, Suneeta was able to explain his dementia as the forgetfulness of old age. To date, no major disruptions had occurred outside their home. Those that transpired within, occasions of disinhibition or incontinence, were managed and hidden from view and as there was no servant or attendant within the home, only Suneeta was aware of these disruptions and cleaned the mess. Thus, due to their geographic location in the middle of a dense suburb, the time they had lived there, Suneeta's affiliation with the local children, her lack of immediate familial support (her mother was dead, she was unmarried and had no siblings), their physical presence on the streets and the mildness of Hari's symptoms, father and daughter wove themselves into the public space of the colony. They were seen as objects of sympathy to be willingly helped by others.

Conversely, those families who were perceived within their communities as caring for a mentally ill or mad family member did experience stigma. The Singhs had long felt the bite of social exclusion. As Harinder Singh's dementia advanced, his family's life had shrunk. Jaspreet, his wife, cared for him while their daughter, Gurneet, managed the housework. The Singhs' son, Ajit, was in his late twenties and of an age and readiness to settle into marriage and children. He was a shy, burly man, who worked in a managerial role in a factory. Usually the family would have faced no more than the usual difficulties of taste and compatibility in finding him a bride. However with Harinder's illness this was not to be. As Jaspreet explained: 'Three to four girls we've approached don't want to marry my son because of his [father's] illness. What the parents are thinking is, "How will our daughter go into that house and manage such a sick person?" This is why they refuse; it's not like the daughters are refusing to marry my son.'

Jaspreet makes two distinctions in this statement: (1) that stigma is based on its perceived link to the labour that will be demanded from the potential daughter-in-law and the polluting effects of this work, rather than on any concern that the disease has a genetic basis; and (2) that stigma functions as a social net, enveloping not just the 'marked' person but also those associated through ties of kinship and love.

Pollution and contagion are inherent risks for carers who perform bodywork. Risk functions metaphorically and instrumentally for cleaning and reaffirming order requires an engagement with disorder and dirt. Those who perform such work operate at the boundaries of containment, risking social propriety, exposing their own bodies and selves in ambiguous ways (Twigg 2000). Faeces, urine, smells and spillages are solids and fluids that cross body boundaries and carers' bodies may often be perceived as contaminated. Matter under fingernails, stains on clothes, lingering odours – these are bodily experiences of dirt and outsiders may feel disgust at seeing such disorder. It threatens the purity of their bodies. Pollution and dirt were lived realities in the Singh home. Harinder was incontinent and the family struggled with his diarrhoea but did not use diapers. Marrying into such a household would render ambiguous the social purity of the bride's identity. This does not refer to gender specific notions of impurity, associated with menstruation or birth, but to the impurities affiliated with those who police the boundary between contagion and boundedness.

When I returned to the Singh home for our second interview, Gurneet – Ajit's sister – had recently quit her job as a school teacher to help her mother run the household. Gurneet was angered by the reaction of outsiders towards their home and at Ajit's difficulty in finding a bride. Alongside her mother and brother, she was part of the family stronghold and again a common narrative of *sevā* and care emerged, punctuated by a lament for the absence of external social support. But as we sat talking in their living room, I noticed Harinder repeatedly attempted to stroke his daughter's leg. Every time his laid his hand on her leg, she stiffened and quietly removed it, placing his hand on his armrest. He would gradually move it back, she would return it – this continued throughout our discussion. She neither complained nor changed her seat nor just held her father's hand. In this small act of body distancing, Gurneet's anger at the rejection of other people was at variance with her own tactics of distancing her father.

The time sensitive and spatial nature of disgust explains this mismatch (Isaksen 2002). For carers such as Gurneet, experiencing the stigma of living within a sequestered household and being angry at other families' unwillingness to send their daughters here, did not preclude her simultaneous resistance to being touched by the source of the stigma, her father. It may be that this was because of her feelings of disgust or her resistance to being touched per se or fear that such touching was sexualized. But she never discussed such sentiments and so this remains conjecture.

Theoretically, disgust is linked to stigma (Miller 1997). Within the household, there are dirty spaces (e.g., the bathroom) and clean spaces (e.g., the kitchen and living room). In transgressing the uses of these spaces, disorderly bodies upset the order of the household and the onus lies with other family members to contain the person. Carers may experience feelings of disgust in doing such work. Their touch may be defined through acts of hygiene, discipline and love in cleaning, bathing and feeding. Caring for a disordered body can entail controlling how that body is touched and in turn, how one lets that body touch oneself. Touching dirt, faeces and urine may be acceptable in a bathing space but not in a living room space. Gurneet may have accepted touching and cleaning her father's faeces and urine in the bathroom, but she could not bear his touch in their living room. In such a way she resented the external stigma from outsiders against her family. But inside, she sought to distance herself bodily from her father.

Loneliness and Space

The experiences of the Singhs were neither acute nor extraordinary. But they were deeply felt and highlight the fact that stigma can often be experienced as small slights, which when compiled can create suffering in everyday life. Other families experienced similar acts of exclusion; Tara, who had dementia, was dismissed from her local park by the other middle-class ladies of her colony; Josie was asked by distant relatives if Su was 'still hanging on'; and Parvati's dinner guests ignored her mother, Meenakshi. There were also reports from ARDSI volunteers in Delhi, Kolkata and Kerala of intense family conflict, dissolved marriages and isolated carers.

This is not to imply that families did not resist stigma. Josie refused further dealings with her relatives, saying she didn't want the kind of compassion they offered, Radha told outsiders that Rajesh's problem was none of their business and Nina frequently told outsiders to 'get lost'. Nina was indignant, '"Hāī bechara, Hāī bechara" (Oh poor thing, Oh poor thing) – what bechara? You've made him like that. This is nonsense! Here I am in control, I can tell people to get lost!'

Moreover, being judged and stigmatized did not preclude families from stigmatizing others nor did it automatically dispel their long-held beliefs. After Tara was dismissed by her peers, her daughter Bhageshwari would send her to the park in the evening with the maid for company. For Bhageshwari the maid was a category rather than a person – 'She doesn't understand that this is a maid and this is somebody' – and sending Tara with the maid was acceptable because Tara was unable to differentiate between maids and people, unlike Bhageshwari who would not have sought social companionship with her maid. Similarly, when I showed Josie photographs of children from the Kamini slum, she muttered 'So many children' in reference to the size of poorer families and Shivbaksh explained that part of the resentment he felt towards his children was because they wouldn't seek his advice when they sought to marry their daughters. Through these vignettes it can be seen that carers were not just victims or martyrs, but people with agency, who were also contradictory, classist and conservative. In short, they were like everybody else – all too human.

Many carers were lonely and did experience suffering because of the stigma associated with mental illness. Suffering was ongoing, mired in domesticities and anchored in everyday illnesses and loss. It was experienced because of stigma that was both internalized and externalized, simultaneously directed to, by and within families. Ajit the rejected groom, Tandon behind his walls, Tara who was dismissed by her neighbours and Shafia and Omar who struggled over community engagement – these are all tales of everyday suffering. Social death may be the end point of stigma, but the journey towards it brings with it exclusion from public spaces and the severance of both small and large ties. Although none of these families were ever socially dead, they did experience increasing loneliness and isolation within themselves and as a family unit.

Loneliness is often equated with anomie, exclusion and marginalization. In the gerontology literature, loneliness has been linked to life expectancy, quality of life and measures of 'successful' ageing (Routasalo et al. 2006; Scharf, Phillipson and Smith 2005; Victor et al. 2000). In the urban studies literature, urban landscapes are seen to be inhabited by an increasingly alienated population influenced by the totalities of capitalism and individualism (Salerno 2003). Loneliness is often premised on the notion of social disconnection, including psychological and sometimes physical distance between family and friends. But loneliness can also happen *in situ*, i.e., within familial relations and domestic places and indeed may sometimes be sought. For this, we need another kind of language, what Coleman (2009) calls, 'being alone together'.

Coleman focuses on homosexuality and desire in an urban restaurant/bar in Delhi. He describes the environment as predominantly a place where people, unknown to each other, could be alone together, survey and watch each other but refrain from any kind of deeper engagement or solidarity politics. These are heterogeneous, anonymous spaces where social solitude is the given norm. People go to places to be alone together. Cinemas and holiday retreats are similar examples. These are predominantly social yet solitary spaces (Coleman 2009).

In trying to extrapolate the connections to my study, let me start with difference: domestic homes are not spaces where unidentified people go to be alone together. They are private areas, different from the anonymity of public urban spaces. These are private social spaces, most often spaces of solidarity and cohesion. People are bound together through characteristics such as kinship, love and culture. They may eat, sleep, relax and live together. In spaces of solidarity, there are family narratives of *sevā* and care. This is the space where children become 'settled', where the good family lives and where normality can be seen.

But the home is also a space for secret stories, hidden gestures and complex, thick connections. Homes contain within them spaces of solitude where people may be strange and unknowable to each other. Specifically, as the dementia progresses, relationships change and people, once familiar, may come to seem foreign. This refers not just to the relationships people with dementia share with their families, but also to how bonds between other family members may be rescripted and rendered strange. Violence, pollution, shifting power relations, new regimes of discipline and pleasure, money and medication may all herald such change. People on the inner may suddenly find themselves on the outer; a powerful father may be undone by his dementia, a mother may be unable to cook, just as a suitable groom is suddenly an unsuitable husband.

Thus changing relationships signaled a loss of power and prestige. Choosing to resist or sequester the family to avoid stigma could result in loneliness. Nina might have exercised agency when she told people to 'get lost', but she also endured loss of friendship and support. Similarly Tandon, in choosing to live in his walled house, was secluded not only from the potentially stigmatizing gaze of his community, but also from the friendships and neighbourliness within his colony.

It is important to emphasize that loneliness was neither linked to intergenerational conflict nor abandonment of close kinship networks. Carers such as Tandon, Nina and Josie all maintained relationships with their children, even though they lived apart. All loved their children. But there were tacit realizations that solitude and loneliness were part of the experience of being the primary carer. These carers did not separate themselves from their families, but the nature of carework made them lonely and emotionally distanced from their families and children. Hence, Nina only asked her son, who lived nearby, for help when she grew 'fed up', just as Tandon conceded, 'Now if I only thought that my children have no time for me then, how can I expect to be a hopeful type?'

The decision to live in solitude was also made by members within the home against each other. Yet, these were silent rebellions and therefore safe. In solitude and lonely spaces, where few could hear and anonymity was assured, unmentionable things could be said without affecting relations within the home. Solitary spaces offered family members a space for their own voice without risking a breakdown in familial cohesion. In solitude people could be unknowable (Rajesh's dementia), say the unspeakable (Rubina's doubts), do the unthinkable (Gurneet's actions) and still be alone together.

Institutional Discriminations

To date there is neither a specific policy on dementia care in India nor sufficient provisions for specific treatment and management practices. In my earlier work (see Brijnath 2008), through an analysis of mental health and ageing legislation and policy, I documented the way in which care was (un)wittingly privatized with the responsibility left largely with the family. In earlier chapters I have shown how this affected families' financial, physical and mental health and their capacity to care.

It was often brought home to me by key service providers that even if there was a policy on dementia care, its implementation would differ significantly from its theoretical ambitions and could never wholly undo what had become standard practice over time. Rather, key service providers emphasized that what would continue to circulate would be an *ad hoc* adherence to notions of rights and care, contingent on environments of deprivation and plenty and individual notions of greed and altruism. Thus, institutional representatives, such as doctors, police and financiers, cared, stigmatized and discriminated against people with dementia and their families according to their own personal politics and assumptions. These varied according to their own status in relation to families' class, gender and income levels (among other factors). The Bhagat's bank, for example, honoured all of Karamjit's cheques even though, by Nina's own admission, his signature had become 'very, very shaky'. As Nina explained, she used their considerable wealth as leverage against the bank: 'I told the bank, "The day you dishonour his cheque I will close my account. If he writes a cheque, you ring me up to confirm it and it has to be allowed, otherwise I will change my account."'

While a determined Nina was able to mobilize financial capital, many others who lacked such substantial wealth could not. ARDSI-DC frequently counselled that following diagnosis, families should immediately organize their finances. This included obtaining a power of attorney, writing wills and property transfers. Those who did not do this could experience difficulty later in accessing accounts. If there was contestation between family members over property, then legal proceedings could go on for decades with no end in sight. India currently has the largest case backlog in the world, with nearly 30 million cases pending (Lal 2008).[1] Property is a particularly sensitive issue and there are numerous stories of usurpation and illegal land grabs. To put this in perspective, there is a group called the *Mritak Sangh*, or Association of the Dead, a north Indian pressure group that campaigns for people who have been declared dead but are still alive and have had their property seized (Fathers 1999).

Older people are seen as especially vulnerable to having their property seized by their children; the tactic of declaring ageing parents insane, then legally taking over their property, has occasionally been used in India (Shah, Veedon and Vasi 1995). Shivbaksh described his youngest son as a *nikāmmā:* (useless, good for nothing) because he had illegally taken *qabza:* (possession) of the back rooms of Shivbaksh's house. The most common advice dispensed by Inspector Tyagi and the Delhi Police was that older people should retain property in their name. The motives behind the recently passed *Maintenance and Welfare of Parents and Senior Citizens Act* (2008) were to protect older people and their assets. The Act mandates that children must care for their parents or risk a fine of Rs 5,000 and/or a jail term of three months. Care is interpreted to mean funds for food, shelter, clothing and medical treatment and parent-child relations may include biological, adoptive and step kin alongside those who might potentially inherit property. One of the architects of the legislation, a major player in a large Indian NGO, admitted: 'You cannot legislate for love and there will always be sceptics. But the thing is we will have to be very prudent and pragmatic because this involves property, this involves money transfers between generations'.

Given that law and money could combine to discriminate against the aged and usurp their rights, property and sanity, any discussion of finances with families had to be carefully broached. Discussions about finances with families where children cared for a wealthy older parent were especially sensitive, for these discussions were framed by this backdrop of property theft and stolen rights. When asked about finances, Nayantara said her father was comfortable, Bhageshwari maintained her mother, Tara, should enjoy her money and Vandhana insightfully pointed out the power dynamics at stake if her in-laws were to be financially dependent on her: 'They are not dependent, they are financially independent . . . So that is a lot because if you're financially also dependent on someone, then it aggravates the situation and in that case I also have an upper hand'.

A medical opinion is required for families to be able to seize property by declaring their aged relative legally insane. The doctor has to deliver a diagnosis of 'mentally incompetent'. If seen as mentally ill, then people with dementia can be placed in asylums, spaces so horrific that even the government wants to shut them down. Without labouring the point, Josie and Su's story from earlier should again haunt us here.

Few age care homes in India will admit people if they are not physically and mentally competent and many have the right to expel residents if their care becomes too burdensome (Lamb 2005, 2009). Hospitals cannot house people with dementia because they are long-term patients. Even if this were possible, there is little awareness amongst care staff of the needs of families and people with dementia. Nandini realized this when her father, S.T. Pillai, was admitted to hospital to have his pacemaker fitted. Ensconced within the medical institution, with its systemic and cultural paradigms, she unsuccessfully tried to communicate with the doctors about her father's dementia. She warned that post-surgery, he would be agitated and confused and needed to be handled appropriately. However, insufficient attention was paid to her concerns and S.T. was viewed by hospital staff as mentally ill. Nandini describes how a surgeon spoke to them in the intensive care unit:

Once the agitation was subsiding, the morning round doctor came. And he stopped and looked at him – I was standing by the bedside – 'Oh you're a psychotic patient, you are a psychotic man, we've got a psychotic man here'. The first time I heard the word 'psychotic' being used and that too, to my father. I didn't say a word. I was just trying to assimilate the word that he used and the emotion that it generates and the diction and his expression when he was using that word.

Health workers' attitudes towards people with dementia and more broadly those with a mental illness, need further explication. With few exceptions (see Jain and Jadhav 2008; Vibha, Saddichha and Kumar 2008), little has been written in India on this. Rather, the focus has mainly been on cultural beliefs and community attitudes to mental health issues. But as Nandini's experience indicates, lack of awareness and insensitive handling of patients and their families colours their interactions and future relationships with health services. This has direct implications for the appropriateness and usability of a service and may also be a contributing factor as to why there is under-utilization of even the limited existing mental health services in India.

In summation, an overview of law, finance and healthcare underscores the fact that in India (1) stigma and discrimination against people with dementia occur largely because they are seen as mentally ill; (2) institutional forces and social processes create a culture in which stigma can travel; (3) the degree of discrimination is linked to perceived differences in power status (influenced by class, gender, etc.); and (4) in practice, institutional representatives are more likely to behave according to the differences in status rather than the policies unless families are able to advocate otherwise.

Conclusion

By describing the moral and social geography of stigma in individual relations, social processes and institutional settings, I have shown how stigma is internalized and externalized. I have also illustrated how stigma is linked to suffering and loneliness, how it informed a project to preserve the normal and how it worked in tandem with institutional forces in law, finance and healthcare. Stigma operated in a different way in each of these moral worlds. In the public spaces of the institution and legislative processes, discrimination was dependent on institutional representatives and the capacity of families to mobilize their financial and cultural capitals. In social processes, pollution, labour and the perceived link to mental illness affected the ability of families to broker successful relationships and marriages. Some families used strategies such as inviting outsiders into the private spaces of their home to 'see' normality within their families and in people with dementia. However, as was demonstrated, this strategy was not without risk.

In each of these moral worlds, stigma flowed alongside existing inequities of power by class, gender and health status. Each moral world also necessitated different tactics to manage stigma. Even within the same moral world, different families used different tactics such as resistance and isolation. Stigma may be a force of cruelty and ill treatment, but is also subtle and accumulative. The careless remarks of a surgeon may not be as cutting as being excluded by friends from the local park. Similarly, what is at stake in social processes may not be as great as what is risked in private spheres. The suffering and loneliness from stigma happens over time and space. While families may feel solidarity in how they respond to stigma, they may also experience solitude in their private homes, where they might whisper their doubts.

In living with stigma, the power relations woven into the institutional and social fabrics of everyday life become visible. Such ties are difficult to unravel because they provide families with the moral and existential frameworks through which to view the world. In trying to respond to stigma and facilitate change there is always the possibility that as power is reshuffled, families may be left worse off than before. This is not to suggest that change is impossible or unattainable – as the stories of carers and families show – but it highlights the fact that it needs to be incremental and gradual. As Parker and Aggleton explain: 'To untie the threads of stigmatization and discrimination that bind those who are subjected to it, is to call into question the very structures of equality and inequality in any social setting . . . [and] to call this structure into question is to call into question the most basic principles of social life' (2003: 18).

Notes

1. To deal with the backlog of cases, since 2001 the Government of India has established over 1,700 'fast track' courts. To date these courts have cleared over 3 million cases. However due to budget cuts the central government announced that it would no longer fund the scheme from March 2011 onwards. As a result, over the past two years, in a number of states, 'fast track' courts have been discontinued (Biswas 2013).

7. THE JOURNEY TO SILENCE

The old *ṭhākur* (lord) lies dying, when his two teenage grandsons are brought before him for the first time. Remorseful for ignoring them all their lives, he now offers the title of his mansion to the sons and their widowed mother. But then the villain, Durjan Singh, arrives to disrupt this delicate reunion. The music changes as he roars at the *ṭhākur*, 'In old age the body becomes useless but you have just rendered your entire life useless!' The ailing *ṭhākur* counters with claims of poison and ruination. A heated exchange follows: Durjan Singh says he has done *sevā* for the *ṭhākur* all his life. '*Sevā*!' scoffs the *ṭhākur*, 'You have tried to kill me at every turn. But I didn't die, maybe because it was the purpose of my life to make sure that these children receive their rights'. Durjan Singh is incensed at the *ṭhākur's* words. '*Khāmosh!*' he cries and there is silence. With this word the balance of power has shifted. The audience gets a sense that the widow, her sons and the old *ṭhākur* are not going to meet a happy end. Durjan Singh confirms this: 'I won't give these beggars one penny. Instead, I'll give you and this family of yours death'.
– *Karan Arjun* (1995)

KHĀMOSH, THE HINDI WORD FOR 'silence', resounds in all its dramatic intensity throughout Bollywood cinematic conflict and symbolizes the power and voice of the speaker to command silence from his/her detractors. '*Khāmosh!*' is often cried in multiple conflict settings, from ageing *ṭhākurs* and land grabs, to angry daughters who battle against conservative fathers. The words flowing on from *Khāmosh!* are heavy in their portent, heralding the detractors' fates until such time as God, true love, revenge or other forces intercede. The word and its context are critical ingredients in the melodrama of Bollywood films. They signal moral conflict, the battle between good and evil, emotional hyperbole, complex kin relations and the epic nature of the story (Ganti 2004).

Following this early scene from the film *Karan Arjun* (1995), Durjan Singh makes good his promise, swiftly dispensing with the ṭhākur and his grandsons, leaving the widow alone in her grief. The widow then pleads with the Goddess Kali to intercede and deliver justice. The murdered boys are reincarnated. They grow up separated from each other and their mother but are reunited twenty years later. They then proceed to take revenge on the ageless Durjan Singh, reclaim their birthrights and live happily ever after. All this is spiced with appropriate song and dance by the brothers and their bosomy beloveds and at different junctures by divine intervention from Kali herself.

Such Bollywood fantasies are *masa:la:* productions, i.e., rather than conforming to particular genres or storylines, they incorporate romance, drama, action, comedy and tragedy into three or more hours. The linearity of the story is unimportant; there are frequent interruptions for songs, subplots and audience intermissions. Lalitha Gopalan (2002) has characterized Bollywood films as a 'cinema of interruptions', wherein the film structure celebrates spatial and temporal discontinuities. Reality and authenticity can also readily be dispensed with. Bollywood filmmakers do not especially focus on facts, instead preferring to offer audiences fantasy and opportunities for imagination and escapism (Ganti 2004).

Taking these key elements of a Bollywood *masa:la:* I analyse the voices of people with dementia. In the place of story and plot logic, there will be romance, comedy, tragedy and action. Poetry and dance will occur in the noisy spaces of the dementia day-care centre and in family homes. The reader will be taken on a flight of fancy, whizzed past representations, ambiguous and open to interpretation, incomplete and complex. Voice is not to be taken as a measure of cognition or memory, typically associated as key indicators of personhood. Instead voice is to be heard as a means of engagement and embodiment of topics such as work, marriage, pleasure, affection and death. These vary by gender and environment and Act 1 of the story will focus on unravelling them.

Like all worthy *masa:la:* productions there will be an intermission, a space to catch one's breath, before moving into Act 2, which will focus on the tragedies of the narrative. The journey to silence will be described – how carers cope when people with dementia advance to the end stages of the disease, how they die and what happens when death finally arrives. Dying is framed by social scripts and political economies; the last section will explain this link between capital and culture.

Some may find it disconcerting that I deliberately do not focus on memory, selfhood and illness, or on how aware people were of being ill or dying. These were inappropriate questions as I quickly learned and risked revealing the diagnosis to the person with dementia and upsetting the family. Any attempts to capture some kind of awareness of memory loss from the person experiencing dementia were often swiftly side-stepped. Through my repeated failures at this task I eventually learned that a predetermined focus on a set of issues does not facilitate listening to what people really want to say. And so, I begin with a brief discussion on selfhood, experience and how I learned to listen.

ACT I

Scene 1: Failures of the anthropologist

The person-centred approach to care has stemmed from efforts by dementia researchers to move away from a medicalized approach to a more personalized social model. In the early 1990s, researchers believed that as the dementia progressed, the self disintegrated until there was nothing left, i.e., a person with dementia became a non-person (Fontana and Smith 1989; Kitwood and Bredin 1992). More recent scholarship challenges such a viewpoint, documenting the discursive praxis in which people with dementia engaged with others to maintain a sense of identity (Beard and Fox 2008; Kitwood 1997; Small et al. 1998; Basting 2009; McLean 2007; Taylor 2008). A key advocate of the latter perspective was the late Tom Kitwood (1997), who argued that neuropathologies and malignant social psychology denied the self of people with dementia and enhanced their suffering. Infantilism, denial, abuse and disregard undermined people's sense of self, excluded them from social life and accelerated their decline. Kitwood's solution was to focus on the person, build meaningful relationships and deliver care and treatment in line with the values and beliefs of the person. He believed that such a person-centred approach could promote quality of life and improve health. There has been mounting evidence from Western countries to support such a claim (see Brooker 2007; Bryden 2005; Nolan et al. 2004).

But Kitwood's approach has also been criticized. The assumption that the self is social and human interaction is essential to construct a sense of self and reality has been challenged. Davis (2004: 377–378) points out that dementia may entail an erosion of selfhood and loss of individual agency that no amount of social interaction can ameliorate. He advocates for greater honesty in acknowledging the violence of the disease and the suffering it creates for people, their families and health workers, rather than sanitizing the dying process through a notion of unimpeachable personhood. Bartlett and O'Connor (2007) point out that the person-centred approach fails to account for the broader socio-political context and loss of citizenship that comes with dementia, relies on others to construct a sense of self for people with dementia and does not sufficiently account for power in caregiving relationships.

Kontos (2006, 2007), while sceptical of Kitwood's model, also problematizes Davis' notion of selfhood, which is premised on cognition and memory. The notion that the self is located only in the mind has its genesis in Western philosophy's Cartesian mind/body split. Yet, as Kontos shows, selfhood also rests in the body and is expressed primordially and socio-culturally. Primordial practices refer to body practices that one does not have to think about in order to perform. A keen seamstress might 'automatically' know how to use the needle and thread or a typist might 'naturally' know where the symbols on the keyboard are. Socio-cultural practices refer to knowledge and appropriate performances of rites and rituals, e.g., saying grace before eating or covering one's head in a temple. Understanding how selfhood is embodied, argues Kontos, must be incorporated into Kitwood's model for there to be truly person-centred care.

In trying to apply all these points in my interactions with people experiencing dementia, the immediate result was often disaster. Despite absorbing the criticisms of the person-centred approach, I hadn't quite understood the point of lived experience and embodiment. In my own self, there was a mind/body split. Ideas around embodiment and person-centred care were stored in some academic corner of my brain while my interactions were transpiring at the level of the body and voice. I was seeking (rather foolishly) a linear interaction: first, somehow establish 'where' people with dementia were in terms of cognition, age, function and memory, and then somehow work to build a relationship.

The first step in this enterprise was to try and determine whether my participants with dementia were mild, moderate or advanced, had difficulty in recalling short- or long-term memories and the extent of their cognitive impairment. I thought I would subtly ask a series of questions, my own version of the Mini-Mental State Examination (Folstein, Folstein and McHugh 1975), as it were. These questions included asking the person with dementia their age, the time of day, location, what they had eaten for lunch, who was the prime minister and how many children they had. In a vague sort of way, I thought from these banal questions some kernel of knowledge would blossom and the key to personhood would suddenly appear. If I was unsure about just what I was doing, my participants were even more befuddled. Those who could still speak rarely did and often looked quizzical; their faces would settle into polite masks of half smiles with confusion in their eyes as I asked them strange questions such as, 'Did you enjoy your lunch today?' There were two notable exceptions – Meera Chopra and Helen Meena Chand – who grew angry with my approach.

When I asked Meera Chopra (80) her age, she indignantly replied, 'What kind of a question is that to ask someone of my age!' When I valiantly pushed on, asking her the time, she grew even more irritated: 'What sorts of questions are these?'

Similarly, Helen Meena Chand, whom I initially assumed could neither walk nor manage daily affairs, stunned me when she proved to be both mobile and capable of passing on messages. I had gone to her home to give her husband, Shivbaksh, the refill script from the Cornwall OPD. When I arrived the front door was wide open and despite repeatedly ringing the bell there was no response. When I began to call out, Helen eventually answered and I followed her voice to her bedroom. Tucked into bed, with the pungent smell of urine permeating the room, she said in a croaky, thin voice, 'He's not at home. He's gone out. I don't know when he will return'. I was reluctant to hand the refill script over to Helen. What if she forgot about it or misplaced it or tore it up? I knew how much these scripts cost in time, effort, money and personal dignity. But with no signs of Shivbaksh returning and my next appointment fast approaching, I gave the script to Helen. Immediately I regretted it. As I attempted to coax it back from her, she became annoyed and suspicious. Her voice grew firm and solid, her speech rapid and incisive: 'Why give me something only to then ask for it back? Why do you want his script anyway? Why should you be the one to put it somewhere else, somewhere safe? What is wrong with leaving the script with me?' I was feeling increasingly stupid and desperate when Shivbaksh suddenly returned. I explained that I had annoyed Helen and he laughed and took the script from her. She cursed me in Haryanvi and Shivbaksh rebuked her in Hindi, '*Arre* she is doing *sevā* for us, working for us and you are giving her *ga:li:* like this?' Helen remained furious, crossed her arms and ignored us both.

Helen's anger at me was justified, as was Meera's irritation. My initial approach was placing them under a psychological microscope. Through some accumulation of facts on age, memory and cognition, I was trying to map their every thought and idea to magically unlock the person within. Being made to feel idiotic was no more than I deserved. Despite reading Nita Kumar's (1992) counsel that just because people are objects of study does not make them simpler, easier, more static or accessible, I blithely made all of these assumptions in my dealings with people with dementia. A most malignant social psychology was at play and though I may now claim to feel embarrassed, at the time any change in my attitude and behaviour was more because of my frustrations, bewilderment and failures. People did not fit into neat clinical categories, there was always ambiguity. Who was Helen? Did she have dementia? At what stage? I remember my field supervisor, Deepak Mehta, counselling, 'Pay attention to voice, listen to what people have to say', and recommending me to read the anthropologist Robert Desjarlais. But in those early days, even listening was hard, because of the novelty and terror of the field. I had to come to terms with the fact that despite knowing the geographic, linguistic and social cues of the city, I did not know my field at all. The anthropologist who is familiar *with* her field does not immediately become familiar *in* her field. I had to learn to live with uncertainty and being overly deterministic was my initial response to cover my anxieties.

There was no fixed event that marked a turning point in my approach. Eventually I just threw up my hands and gave up trying to establish who the person was or how old they thought they were. I just began to be with them. Time, space and personhood were pushed aside. In its place emerged a phenomenological understanding. This change was driven by lived experience, intellectually and bodily. In the early January days of fieldwork, when I was busy pigeonholing people and the Delhi traffic roared in my ears, the dust made my fingers prune and my feet crack and peel relentlessly. By the end of April, at once more and less familiar with the world, the rising heat, dust and chaos of the city had browned me, straightened my hair and strengthened my limbs.

At the same time, my dealings with people with dementia grew more fluid and touching became the most common way to engage. I often found myself holding hands with people, stroking their hair and rubbing their backs. With women, blowing kisses and hugs were permissible; with men such behaviour was inappropriate. People responded positively to shows of affection and these were some of my sweetest encounters in the field. We danced, sang and talked to each other. These experiences were shaped by the slow loss of language and function among my participants and a different attuning of my listening and observation skills. Thus, through my body and experience, I learned first-hand of what Merleau-Ponty wrote long ago:

> The real is a closely woven fabric. It does not await our judgement before incorporating the most surprising phenomena, or before rejecting the most plausible figments of our imagination . . . The world is not an object such that I have in my possession the laws of its making; it is the natural setting of, and field for, all my thoughts and all my explicit perceptions (1945 [2007]: 136–137).

Interruption: The Dance

Cut to a scene in the dementia day-care centre in Kochi, Kerala. Chanchala (80), small, thin and dark with a near shorn head, wears a vermillion blouse and white cotton sari. She is sitting down and as I walk past her, she stretches her hand towards me. I take it and we wander over to another set of chairs. She does not sit down; instead she holds both of my hands and I gently swing them from side to side. She follows my movements, still holding onto my hands and we are swinging our hands together. Then I gently shake my hips from side to side and Chanchala follows me. Now we are dancing to silent music. A few staff members notice and giggle. Eventually I stop and when I lead Chanchala to her seat she sits down. I blow her a kiss and she raises her hand to her lips, kisses it, then cups my cheek and my chin with that hand and looks into my eyes. Whether a connection is made or Chanchala is naturally affectionate to everyone remains unclear. Later in the ARDSI bus, she will not tolerate my back to her. She repeatedly touches me on my shoulder and when I turn to face her, she blows kisses. If I focus on anyone else, she touches my shoulder and demands attention and affection.

Scene 2: Men at Work

Robert Desjarlais (1997), in his work with homeless people in Boston, wrote about the difficulties of representation when narrative and experience were disrupted and disjointed. Trying to develop a cohesive story, 'tying things together through time', rests on novelty, continuity, transformation, plot and movement. But for those who struggle, whose days are defined by contingency, illness, medication and marginalization, such characteristics do not apply. In its place, according to Desjarlais, a critical phenomenology is necessary, one that ties together how people think, feel and experience things and the processes by which they come to pass (1997: 22–25). Such a phenomenology is political because it is concerned not only with the modalities of experience but also with the way in which the forces of politics, economics and culture come to shape these experiences. Given that 'experience is the medium through which people engage with the things that matter most to them, both individually and collectively' (Kleinman and Fitz-Henry 2007: 54), it is necessary to understand this dialectic between and within people, in the complex but ordinary routines of everyday life.

In my sample, in Delhi, people with dementia led boring lives. Their days consisted of routines defined by others: prayer times, bathing time, mealtimes, siestas, evening walks and bed. In between there were many hours in which no activities were undertaken and people sat in chairs or lay in their beds. Carers often used this time to do paid work and housework or to rest. Depending on the mood, capacity and interest of carers and people with dementia, sometimes activities such as peeling vegetables (n=3), reading and writing (n=4), watching TV (n=3) or listening to music (n=5) were undertaken. With the exception of Nina who tried to fill Karamjit's days with as many activities as possible, most carers were too preoccupied with the basic activities of daily living to pay much attention to anything else.

This left people with dementia with few opportunities for pleasure or occupation. Boredom created too much time that was spent by slowly waking up and getting dressed, protracted prayers and lying down. Many felt depressed and oscillated from being withdrawn and quiet to aggressive and repetitive. Rajesh Menon (71) was depressed and bored because he could not work:

> Actually after retirement I was offered a job. But these people (his family), they did not allow.
> *Would you like to work?*
> Yes, I can spend time – not for money. I can spend time.
> *Occupy yourself?*
> Yes. I can spend time. Engage.

For Rajesh, time was a commodity in surplus. He wanted to spend it in occupying his mind in a way that was meaningful to him. He had been an accounts officer and worked all his life to provide for his family. Having retired over a decade ago and following his dementia diagnosis, his life had profoundly changed. His wife, Radha, cared for him and they lived with their daughter, son-in-law and two grandchildren in a small flat in west Delhi. While Radha's days were full with caring for Rajesh and her grandchildren, Rajesh's routine was relatively empty. He was depressed and disengaged, spending much of his time reading the paper, watching TV or napping. He rarely left his home, had few friends to visit and constantly hankered for his 'native place' in Kerala.

Rajesh was not the only man who saw work as a means of engagement and greater self-esteem. There were many other men with dementia whose careers were imprinted in their bodies and central to their identity. Ex-military man, Kaalathinnu, was crisp and contained in his movements. He never slouched in his seat, his shirt was ironed, his clothes unstained and he was focused on order and discipline. Similarly Francis and Santosh were 'men at work' in the ARDSI dementia day-care centre in Kochi. Francis, a former clerk of the High Court, enjoyed his days at the 'department' and officiously signed all newspapers, while Santosh, an erstwhile salesman for a powder company, still touted his 'product' in the day-care centre.

Even those who disliked work could not escape it. Moses (79), despite retiring, still spent his days 'at work' as an 'assistant' at the day-care centre, constantly trying to get leave. He had written a sheaf of letters to the day-care manager asking for a holiday. His letters were mostly a jumble of his name and former occupation; often he was his own referee. Intrigued by his request, I approached him at the end of the day:

> *I've read your application for leave*
> [Remains silent, listening]
> *I think it is a good idea. Take holiday tomorrow* [Tomorrow is Sunday and the day-care centre is closed]
> [Nods]
> *Yes, now is a good time [to take leave]. We are not so busy*
> *Yes, it can be adjusted later*
> *Yes, no problem. Is that ok with you Moses?*
> Yes [walks away].

Globally, while there may be many kinds of masculinity, income generating work has tended to be a critical component of hegemonic masculinities (Connell 1995; Fitzsimons 2002). In the Indian subcontinent, in dominant and subaltern forms of masculinity, men are perceived as the primary breadwinners (Jackson 1999). Employment is a source of identity and power within the public sphere and the household, offering men the respect of their peers and power and control over their wives and children. Paid work is also a means by which male dominance over the public sphere is retained and has been linked to nationalist discourses (Chatterjee 1990; Gupta 2002). Whereas a hegemonic feminine identity can be achieved through caring, childbearing and/or paid work, for men, loss of employment signals loss of power and self. Unemployment is a point of 'crisis', signalling transformations in gender roles and relations (Haque and Kusakabe 2005; Radhakrishnan 2005). For these men with dementia, work was written into their bodies. Their desire to be 'at work', sign papers, sell products, move authoritatively and even apply for leave, were attempts to hold onto power, to pass time in a meaningful way and to anchor themselves in what was familiar in a changing world. Being at work mitigated the losses associated with ageing, retirement, diminished bodily function, lessened status within the home and the slow removal of personhood as a result of these changes.

In addition to work, men also sought to anchor their identities in the personal achievements of others. In the Bhagat family home, Karamjit took my hand and guided me around, pointing to each cross-stitched framed picture. I did not know until then that Nina had sewn all of these pictures and Karamjit wanted to ensure that I noted that down. Up until that point I knew Nina was engaged in a struggle to preserve Karamjit's identity, but I now realized that his identity was inextricably fused to hers. Just as Nina had said, 'I think that if a man loses his identity he is lost. What has he got

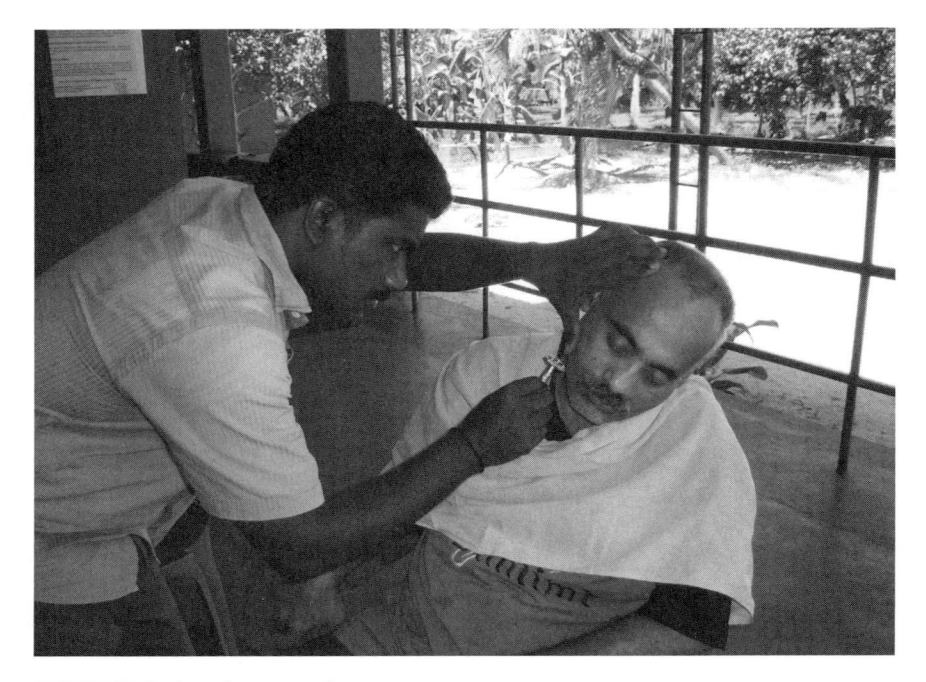

FIGURE 7.1 An afternoon shave

left if I am not known as Nina Bhagat?', so too Karamjit took pride in his wife's accomplishments, showing them off to visitors in their home.

Alongside the intimacies of personal relations, pleasure was also to be had through engaging in private activities publicly. In the ARDSI dementia respite care centre in Guruvayoor, Kerala, shaving was an activity that most male residents enjoyed. In the afternoon, a male staff member would arrive on the porch with a brush, mug, lather and razor. The residents would lie in their chairs dozing as he would shave each of them in turn. In a gesture of extreme trust, they would lay with their heads back, keep their eyes closed and leave their jugulars exposed. For them this was an act of great pleasure. Most would rest their arms on their stomach. Even noisy, disruptive residents were quiet during their shave (see Fig. 7.1).

Experiences such as shaving or showing off a spouse's accomplishments speak to Marriott's (1976: 111) famous observation of 'dividual' selves in the subcontinent. According to Marriott, persons in South Asia are not so much individual, self-contained units but are dividual or divisible. They absorb heterogeneous and material influences and simultaneously put out their own body substance codes, i.e. essences or residues of themselves. In this way, people are absorbing and incorporating each other into their notion of self, exchanging and circulating substance codes.

When the experience of dementia care is added, with the attendant intimate exchanges of bodily substance codes that such care entails, a second layer of dividuality is operationalized. Activities such as shaving, working and taking pride in a life partner's achievements become ways in which people reproduce within themselves elements of each other in a common social context. Therefore, just as with dementia care there may be dirt and matter out of place, so too there are constant efforts to emplace and embody within people with dementia and their carers those key aspects of identity and personhood that really matter to them.

Interruption: The Poem

> Mid pleasures and palaces though we may roam,
> Be it ever so humble, there's no place like home;
> A charm from the sky seems to hallow us there,
> Which, seek through the world, is ne'er met with elsewhere.
> Home, home, sweet, sweet home!
> There's no place like home, oh, there's no place like home!
> – *Home, Sweet Home*, John Howard Payne (1823)

I am talking to Parvati Gowda, who cares for her mother, Meenakshi. 'Yesterday she asked me, "Where are we going?"' and, Parvati replied, 'Home, sweet home'. Then Parvati said the first line of the poem – 'Mid pleasures and palaces though we may roam'. Meenakshi hears it and then she recites the rest of this poem, all five verses and thirty lines in perfect iambic pentameter.

Scene 3: Bride and Prejudice

Women with dementia also struggled with loss, but their foci were domesticity, beauty, poetry and children. As their lives grew increasingly uncertain, efforts were centred on preserving and building relations in the home. Women often harassed their daughters and husbands to let them cook, care for their children and socialize with visitors by serving them tea. Notions of femininity and the power of women within the home framed these practices. Mrs Hamdari had been the matriarch of her family for many years. But as her dementia progressed, her duties and caring responsibilities were transferred to her daughters. Her younger daughter, Nayantara, explained to me that her mother often acted out her frustration by resisting the changes:

> She is a very caring person and she can't help her [motherly] nature, so it was very difficult, very difficult. She has gone through not feeling in command, not handling the house or herself but slowly, slowly this is becoming less of an issue. Initially there was lots and lots of aggression and a lot of fighting about wanting to cook. She used to be a fantastic cook but now we don't let her cook. When my younger sister was here from America, she got the flu and five times in the night she [mother] woke up and went to check on her. She was very concerned.

Veena Das has argued that Indian women experience their bodies as both object and subject, in that gender is scripted onto the body and its images, as well as played out within everyday relations in public and private spaces (1988: 193). Mrs Hamdari's attempts to cook, care for her daughter and socialize can be understood as an embodiment and enactment of gender scripts that also play out in everyday kin relations. Home is central to this dynamic because for older Indian women home can sometimes be an uncertain location. Compared to their male peers, widows in north India tend to be economically and politically marginalized and to experience greater levels of neglect and abuse, poorer health and higher mortality (see Agarwal 1998; Chen and Dreze 1995). Given that older women have an increased likelihood of having their property stolen from them and being forced to retreat elsewhere, home is a space that literally represents the stakes of power, emotions and economics. For women in my sample, home occupied a strong place in their mind. Helen Meena Chand and Meera Chopra rarely left their homes even to see doctors. In contrast, Lakshmi Kumari continuously hankered after her home in Pakistan and Meenakshi Ranjarajan harassed her daughter to take her to her childhood home in Kerala.

While home represented security and domesticity, it was not just aligned with traditional notions of family and care. The home was also a space for beauty and consumption. This duality is an extension of the representation of urban Indian women in popular culture; just as women are presented in the nexus of tradition and modernity, so too are their homes. Independence, glamour and consumption lie on one side, conservative family values and middle-class nationalism on the other (Thapan 2001). Though much of the literature has tended to examine this dynamic in the lives of younger and middle-aged women, older women also occupy this juncture (Deshpande 1998; Dube 1988; Narayan 1997; Thapan 2000). As the dementia loosened her inhibitions, Gauri (75), widowed with adult children and grandchildren, had become increasingly obsessed with finding a suitable husband. To her, a husband represented income for her dreams of a wealthy home, which included cars, bungalows and many servants:

How do I seem to you? Am I beautiful? Will I get a boy?
Yes, you seem very beautiful and good to me. Of course you will get a boy, why not?
Best, best, doctor or engineer, nothing else.

To secure a suitable husband, Gauri sought to trade her beauty for wealth. Her notion of beauty centred on her fair skin. This was a running joke in the ARDSI day-care centre in Kerala, where many of the attendants were darker skinned. The bus driver of ARDSI's van would tease Gauri by asking her what her name meant: 'It means brightness', she replied. 'No, it means darkness', he teased. '*Arre sala* (oh bastard), it means whiteness, you're the black one', she retorted.

Gauri's association between whiteness and beauty is a common one in India, one that has been increasingly capitalized on by multinational cosmetic companies through their skin-whitening products, Bollywood stars and online matrimonial agencies (Osuri 2008). In India, beauty is whiteness, tied to hetero normative patriarchal orders and higher classes and castes. Bollywood has played a key role in disseminating this image both in India and transnationally, a strategy that has colonial roots, invokes traditional notions of femininity and reinforces existing power relations (Reddy 2006). In a middle-class Indian zeitgeist, whiteness represents a safe and readily marketable form of beauty that women can apply to or mobilize from their bodies to lever themselves into higher socio-economic positions. In a private moment, in her afternoon repose, Gauri quietly tells of a life hard lived, of days spent cleaning, scrubbing, studying and raising children. 'My parents said I had to try to do everything otherwise I would make nothing of myself', she says. Gauri's tactics can thus be seen as an effort to accrue more status and power within the wider context of patriarchal inequities and political and economic marginalization.

INTERMISSION

A person's body dies but not their spirit, not their life.
I am a spirit, I am not a body.
Once this body is worn out I will discard it.
But I am limitless, just like God is limitless.
I will keep coming back.
Now in this life I have had it the best – I have been a man.
In my next life I could come back as a bird, a tiger, a snake,
I have attained *mukti*; the body is such a thing.
– Kundan Lal Chopra

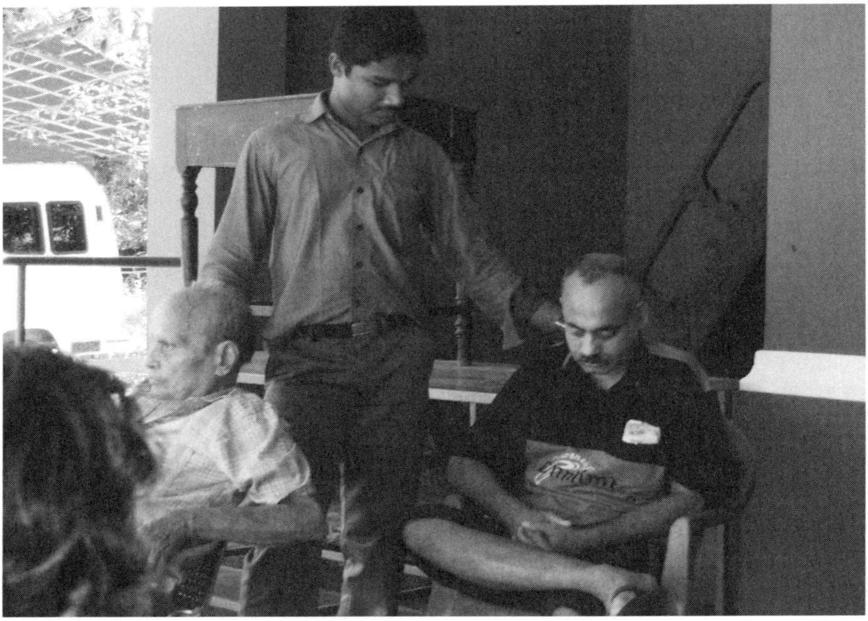

FIGURE 7.2 An afternoon nap

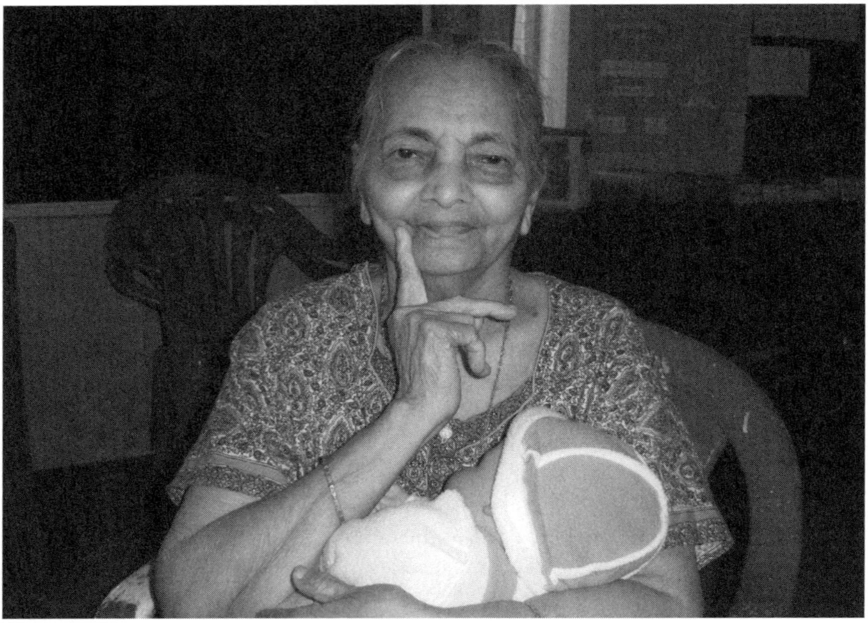

FIGURE 7.3 Beautiful Gauri

THE JOURNEY TO SILENCE *171*

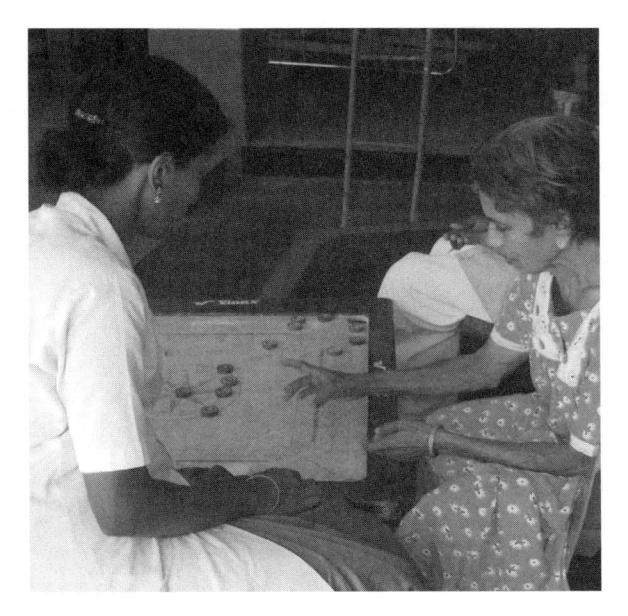

FIGURE 7.4 Playing carom

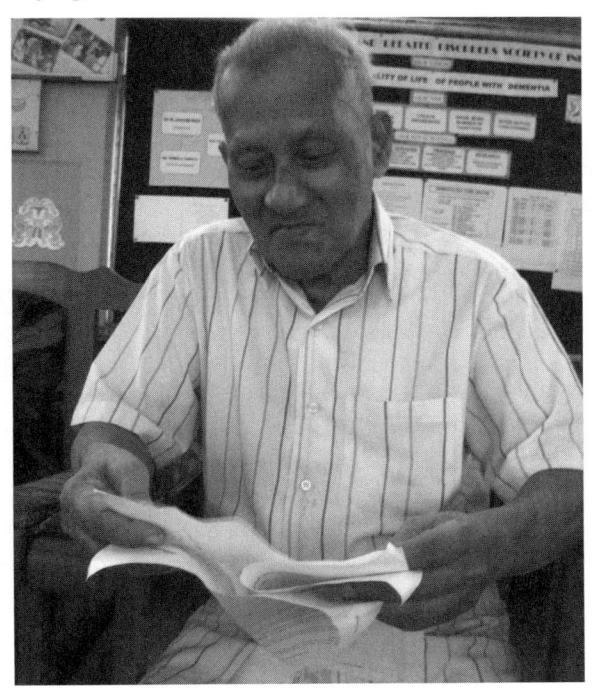

FIGURE 7.5 Men at work

ACT II

Scene 1: 'It's easy to let go now'

With time, people with dementia began to lose function. They forgot how to walk, talk, swallow, turn, go to the toilet and eventually consistently failed to recognize their own family members. In order to manage these degenerations, the efforts of the carers' increasingly centred on diet, exercise and medication. Though families incurred significant costs for such interventions, they were sought nevertheless and no one considered palliative care. Families were disinclined to withdraw the feeding tube or not use the ventilator. The inextricable link between a carer's sense of self, the need to try all forms of an *ilāj* and to give the greatest amount of *sevā*, made the moral stakes too risky for such decisions.

In contrast some people with dementia sought non-intervention and death. Rajesh Menon spent all his time harassing his wife, Radha, to return to their 'native place' in Kerala. When asked why, Rajesh replied:

> I like Trivandrum. I want to be in Trivandrum. I want to be (sic) peaceful death there.
> *You want to be peaceful there?*
> Peaceful death in Trivandrum.

Like Rajesh, Helen also wanted to die. When I visited her home for my second interview with Shivbaksh, I asked her how she was. 'I am ready to go up', she responded. Talking about wanting to die and planning for death have been noted in other studies on ageing in India. Sarah Lamb (2000), in her work with Mangaldihi villagers in West Bengal, found that it was common for older people to plan and discuss their death. Lawrence Cohen (1998) describes how those who were *marnevālā* (about to die) were regarded by Varanasi residents as people who had lost their authority and were doing *bakbak* (prattle; chatter). Similarly, in my study, though people with dementia expressed a desire to die, their carers often dismissed such talk and concentrated their efforts on preserving life. This did not mean denial or lack of preparation for death. Indeed, because death was inevitable, many strived to fulfil the wishes of their ill loved one. Radha did take Rajesh back to Kerala for short breaks, Shivbaksh gave Helen all the *biːɽiːs* she wanted to smoke and Lakshmi Kumari's family took her to visit her hometown in Pakistan.

Fighting to the end was part of *sevā* even though, as Josie pointed out, 'It's easy to let go now'. Families caring for people who were in the late stages of dementia underwent their own emotional metamorphosis as their loved one declined. They tried to limit their emotional attachments towards their loved ones and avoided thinking about the end, while stoically accepting the inevitable. Shafia, married for over twenty-five years to Omar, had spent the last seven years caring for him. With Omar on a feeding tube, ill and near death more than once, Shafia knew it was a matter of time. Even as she feared the financial stresses of widowhood, she prepared herself for Omar's death:

> Comfort and consolation – you have to be ready. This is the way it is for us. This is the way it is for everyone because life and death are in God's hands and there is nothing we can do. This is our fate and it rests with Allah. When a man is in his condition, when he can't stand, how long is he going to live with this illness? He can't eat, he drools, his *hāth-pair* don't work. You have to endure this; you have to prepare yourself.

Interruption: Journal entry, 28th August 2008

When I called Shivbaksh this morning, after days of trying, I was surprised by the disorientation, grief and loneliness in his voice. 'How is Helen?' I ask.

> She has gone to her *shmasha:n* (cremation).
> [Gasps] *She's dead?*
> Yes.
> *Can I come visit you tomorrow?*
> Yes come.
> *What time?*
> Come anytime, I just sit at home alone these days.

Scene 2: 'My heart is cut on the inside, my heart weeps'

During my time in Delhi three people died – Surinder Dharam Singh (58), Helen Meena Chand (82) and Gautam Mukherjee (88). A year before I interviewed Namita Sood, her mother had died, aged 83. Their voices were now silent. Their last days were some of the most emotional and labour intense days of caring for their families as the forces of medicine, capitalism and culture came to bear on them.

In my study, people with dementia, by virtue of their middle and elite class status and urban locale, tended to spend their last days in the hospital. They were often admitted for fevers, pneumonias, hip fractures and blood infections. Very few died in their homes and often these deaths were sudden. Gautam Mukherjee had a high fever for two days and died in his sleep before his scheduled admission to hospital the following morning. In contrast, Helen Meena Chand had a fall, fractured her hip and was admitted to hospital. There she contracted an infection, experienced a loss of appetite, lapses in consciousness and eventually began to excrete and vomit blood. In her final two days, she went on the ventilator and twenty-five days after her admission she died alone in the early hours of the morning.

In comparing these two cases, there is a need to actively avoid the easy conflation of 'good' and 'bad' death. Such an approach risks elevating specific cultural scripts around dying to universal categories, often at the expense of other cultural ideas around dying. Anthropologist Susan Long comparing Anglophone countries (such as US, Britain and Australia) and Asian nations (such as Japan) found that though choice, place, timing and personhood were common features of a 'good' death, their interpretations and applications were quite different (See Table 7.1). However, extending these findings to the Indian context must be made with caveats for such scripts hold greater sway in relation to urban, middle-class and elite Indians who are already engaged with biomedicine. The poor and those in rural areas often evince and experience very different cultural mores informing the dying process.

In applying the findings from Table 7.1 to my study participants it can be seen that Gautam Mukherjee's death was not necessarily 'good' just because he died at home, just as Helen's was not 'bad' because it occurred in a hospital. If not for his sudden passing, Gautam too would have been in hospital. Being in hospital did not negate 'goodness' and other families described positive interactions with hospital staff that helped to facilitate 'good' deaths. Nursing staff telephoned the Sood family at 4 A.M. to come and say goodbye to their mother. Namita recalled:

> When we went into the room she opened her eyes and she smiled such a beautiful smile. We said her prayers and to the last strains of the *Gāyatrī-Mantra*, she slipped away. When we brought her back home and washed her, no rigor mortis set in; when you saw her face, it was a smile, it was a really beautiful smile. She [grew up] in a Sikh orphanage and she died around 4–4:15 A.M. The Sikhs say this is *ammrit-vela:* [ambrosial period] – it is the most beautiful time to go.

Through Namita's story, a 'good' death is socially constructed: her mother was alert and smiling, she was surrounded by her family, her favourite prayers were recited and she died at an auspicious time. The 'good' death was even embodied, as there was no rigor mortis and Mrs Sood had a smile on her face in death. By now it should be evident that few practices in India strictly obey boundaries of caste, class, religion and

TABLE 7.1 Comparing cultural scripts on dying in Anglophone and Asian countries

	Anglophone countries	Asian countries
Choice	Patient and families follow the advice of physicians but there is a common ideology that the patient in consultation with the family decides when and how to die.	Patient and families strongly follow the advice of physicians. Also strong emphasis on god as decision maker, e.g., 'it's in God's hands now'.
Place	Strong preference for death to occur at home surrounded by family.	Preference among the middle class for death to occur in hospitals, surrounded by family.
Timing	Person should die when the situation is hopeless and there is no longer any point to prolonging life.	Person should die when they are old and have lived a full life. There should be efforts made to prolong the life of younger people, even if the situation is hopeless.
Personhood	The person should be aware and in control of their faculties, i.e., they should not be a 'vegetable'.	Focus is on the relationship between the person and the social world even beyond death.

Adapted from Long (2004: 913–928).

gender. The Soods, who were Hindu, borrowed from Sikh precepts to comfort themselves, reflecting the cross-pollination, amalgamation and re-interpretations of ideas and customs as they circulate amongst different communities.

Hindu ideals around dying in India, particularly for men, see the body as a sacrifice to be made on the funeral pyre. Death is to happen in old age, following a life replete with children and grandchildren. In the days leading up to death, the dying man is meant to forgo food and consume only water in order to weaken his body, so that the 'vital breath' may leave it more easily and to purge himself of faecal matter to purify himself. Then, having set his affairs in order and surrounding himself with his family, the man not so much dies as relinquishes life and his body (Parry 1981). Those whose intention to sacrifice themselves through death has not been established (e.g., children or those who meet violent and unnatural ends), or who are unfit sacrifices because of their sins, or whose death is already seen as an offering to the gods (e.g., ascetics), are not permitted to be cremated. Instead they are to be immersed either in water or earth (Das 1976).

When viewed from this standpoint, even deaths such as Helen's, which may seem 'bad', have 'good' elements. She had lived a full life with children, grandchildren and great-grandchildren, her body was purified leading up to her death and she set her affairs in order before dying. Shivbaksh recalled that prior to going onto the ventilator, she recognized him, sat up and put her arms around him. Even 'bad' deaths have redeeming features, just as 'good' deaths have negative elements that people choose not to dwell on. Thus, to definitively categorize deaths as 'good' or 'bad' bleaches out their ambiguities and glosses over the embedded moralities in the cultural scripts that surround dying in India.

With death, some families observed traditional funeral rites according to their religion, while others opted for a more pragmatic line. Shilpi Mukherjee electrically cremated Gautam and did not await the arrival of her sons from overseas to fulfil any last rites; Shivbaksh observed all the Hindu ceremonial funeral rites for Helen. Even here the reasons for such practices were motivated by cosmic and earthly concerns: Namita Sood's mother had wanted a no-fuss electrical cremation but at the time of her death, electricity shortages in Delhi were so acute that there was no guarantee the body would be fully burnt. Rather than risk a half burnt body being dumped somewhere, Mrs Sood's daughters observed all the rites and burnt their mother's body with wood.

Irrespective of attitudes towards funeral rites, photos of the deceased assumed a central role in families' homes. Enlarged, laminated portrait pictures of the deceased were placed on living room mantlepieces or on prayer altars in bedrooms. Sometimes lights and garlands were placed around these photos and the sacred *tikka* might be applied to the portrait's forehead. The photos tended to show the person a few years prior to their death, with the exceptions of Su and Gautam whose pictures showed much younger, stronger, more virile versions of themselves. Commemorating deceased family members through photos is customary across Indian society and is a way to 'extend lineage continuity beyond the lives and transient memories of living family members' (Lamb 2000: 177). The photo functions spatially and temporally to link the deceased elder to future generations, who will venerate them. Photos allow an imagined connection to be made between the divine and everyday worlds through the elder who has attained *mukti* (release) but continues to be remembered within the bonds of kinship and family (Lamb 2000).

Death also brought more immediate emotional and geographic changes to carers' lives. Soon after Gautam's death, Shilpi Mukherjee's sons began to make preparations to take their widowed mother back to the US to live with them. Josie's daughter came to live with her for six months and Namita Sood and her sister returned to work. For Namita, who found the caring experience very positive – 'It was seven years of picnic for us' – the picnic was now over. And while these carers grieved – they all acknowledged that they had prepared themselves for this moment – there was one exception – Shivbaksh Chand.

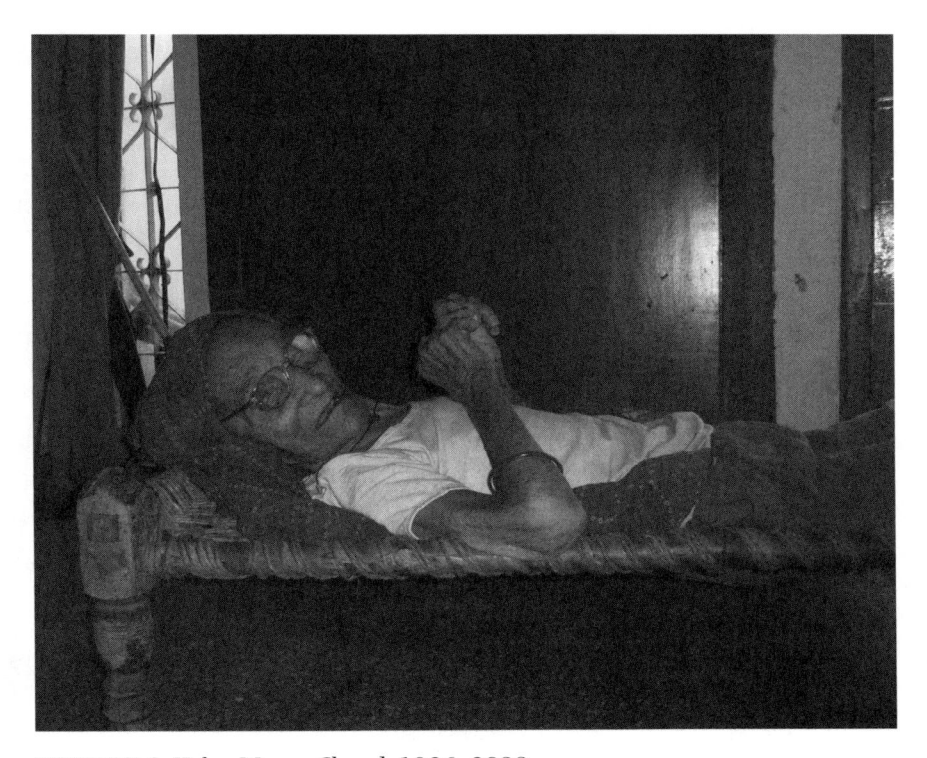

FIGURE 7.6 Helen Meena Chand, 1926–2008

Shivbaksh had felt the cut of change most deeply. All through the months when Helen was alive (Fig. 7.6), he was jocular, loud, irascible and cheeky. He had filled their home with the noises of cooking, television and visitors. When I first met him in February he had on a white full-sleeved *kurta:-pajama*. But as the days grew warmer and Helen became frailer, on each subsequent occasion, Shivbaksh seemed to wear less and less. In our last meeting, he had on a white vest and shorts and had lost weight. Whereas before he would hold forth on his sofa and punctuate his speech with explosive hand gestures, now he had retreated to a corner near his front door with a newspaper. Gone was the wild waving of his arms. The disciplinary ties in his life had also loosened; he admitted to drinking to excess and, when his mind was totally k͟harāb (ruined), to smoking. There was neither talk of his dementia nor of visits to the OPDs. He rarely went to meet his friends at the local dispensary across his street. Instead he was quiet, contemplative, sadly awaiting his own death: 'It could happen anytime and everyone has to go. A human being is born alone and must die alone. It is my time to die, I've lived my life'.

Scene 3: The Political Economy of Dying and Organ Donation

Although there has been a large amount of work written on funeral rites and customs in India (see Das 1976, 1998; Madan 2004; Mines 1989; Orenstein 1970; Parry 1981, 1985; Schmalz 1999), little has been published on the political economy of dying and dementia. Sharon Kaufman (2006), based on her work in American hospitals, illustrates the difficulties in decision making when dementia is accorded the value 'near death' and the disputes that arise when hospital staff and family members disagree over that value. Kaufman, through her analysis, shows that decisions to prolong or end life are moral choices that result from medical categorizations, institutional imperatives and deliberations about value.

In India, when people die within institutional settings such as hospitals, medical interventions and the value of life are also linked to capital. Medical interventions are bound to ideas of *sevā* and families' efforts to resist dying are part of the dying process. This applies even to those for whom there is little hope. Often people who were terminally ill were put on ventilators to prolong their life. P.K. Singh, a volunteer at ARDSI in Delhi, describes the last days of his wife who had Alzheimer's disease:

> I had to put my wife in the hospital because of an emergency. She got high fever and an infection in her lung. There they said, 'We'll have to put her on a ventilator'. Putting her on a ventilator had two implications. Firstly, it is very expensive. It is about Rs 11,000–Rs 12,000 a day. And the second thing is, once you put it on, then you cannot take it off. It is a life support system. There is also some legal issue and you can't take it off. It has to be there until the patient is brain dead. Then the doctors decide that they can remove it.

Class is implicit in such a paradigm, for only those who can afford to pay for ventilators and life prolonging treatments are able to avail themselves of these options. This goes to the politics and value of unequal lives and fits within a larger issue of health service delivery in inequitable settings. Das and Hammer (2004) note that private providers in Delhi tend to over-medicate and/or perform unnecessary procedures for cash incentives, while public providers are more likely to under-treat or insufficiently treat patients (who are typically poor). Specifically with older patients who are dying, the cultural reluctance to end life even in terminal cases such as P.K'.s wife, determines medical interventions, as do politico-economic forces such as money, access and the values assigned to the lives of the rich and poor.

Nowhere perhaps are these disparities more evident or contrary than in organ donation. In death, Namita Sood and Josie Dharam Singh attempted to donate Mrs Sood's and Su's body respectively. But these efforts failed due to the misalignment of medical categorizations, institutional imperatives and deliberations about value. Before I explicate these links, a brief detour into the values around organ donation is necessary.

Donation has an ambiguous value in India for two reasons: (1) it evokes a tripartite social relationship between donor, recipient and the nation-state; and (2) has a murky association with organ trafficking. On the one hand, organ donation can be seen as an act of 'ethopolitics', what Nikolas Rose (2001: 18) characterizes as the ways in which the 'ethos of human existence ... have come to provide the "medium" within which the self-government of the autonomous individual can be connected up with the imperatives of good government'. Public appeals to donate eyes, organs, or blood as the gift of sight or of life or sustenance, draw on discourses of class, nation and immortality. The most famous Indian advertisement for eye donation in the 1990s featured the newly crowned Miss World, Aishwarya Rai, offering to 'Leave my eyes when I die and have someone see again, to look at our world through *my* eyes long after I'm gone' (emphasis added). Since then many celebrities, film stars, cricketers and politicians have pledged their organs after their death. Popular slogans and advertisements to boost organ donation – 'Life . . . Pass it on!' 'Organ donation, the gift that lives on' – suggests a vision of immortality, as one's life is never truly gone but merely transferred into another body. Much like the photos of the deceased in families' homes imagine a link between the divine and the everyday, so too organs are mobilized as new kinds of commemorative objects. Photos may occupy prime position in a living room, but organs live in the body.

Additionally organ donation is mobilized to venerate the nation and its institutions through the donation of blood and bodies from its citizenry. Mass drives for blood donation have been tied to politically commemorative events such as the death anniversaries of assassinated politicians and ideas of national integration (Copeman 2004, 2009). Cadaver donation is marketed as an ascetic practice to further the knowledge of medical institutions (Copeman 2006). Thus, through blood and body parts, complex social continuities are imaged between deceased and recipient and between donors and the nation-state.

But the principles of this new biomorality are undermined by a reality of low organ donation, surpluses of organ trafficking and stories of desperation, coercion and exploitation of the poor while the elite purchase and use such body parts. In this new biosocial enterprise, as the relationship between India's poorer and wealthier citizens is literally re-embodied, 'Whatever the relation, if any, between buyer and seller, the dominant vision of biosociality has shifted from the utopian . . . into a *dual economy* of sacrifice and substance' (Cohen 2001: 20).

Within this uncertain terrain of values, Namita and Josie's efforts at etho-politics also encountered institutional bureaucracies and poor resources. Because Mrs Sood died outside business hours, the organ banks could not be contacted to harvest her body. In addition, as she had died in August, the Sood family could not delay her cremation for risk of putrefaction in the heat. As Namita explained:

> Those organ fellows were terrible because you couldn't get in touch with them. Otherwise she [would have] donated her brain and the rest of her organs. They should have a twenty-four-hour service because it doesn't come from higher on that you're going to die in office hours.

Josie tried to be more organized in her approach to donation but still failed. On his final admission to the hospital, Su had pneumonia and could no longer swallow. Realizing that the end was near, Josie initiated conversations between herself, ARDSI and Dr Yashaswini to try and donate Su's organs. Yashaswini advised shifting Su to her hospital because of the difficulties associated with moving deceased persons (apparently ambulances cannot transport deceased persons and private taxis charge considerably more to do so). Also she cautioned Josie about the condition that Su's body would be in when it was returned to her: dissections and organ retrievals often led many families to reject the body post harvesting. These procedures left Josie unsure about whether to donate as she described the doctors as, 'All ready with their knives'.

But a few days later when Su died, Josie took the decision to donate his body. The Autopsy Unit then refused to accept his body, claiming that because Su had Alzheimer's disease, nothing could be harvested. Then the Organ Donation Unit from the same hospital said that Su's eyes could be used and that they were on their way; forty-five minutes later the same call and message were relayed to the family. The family waited for nearly four hours but nobody arrived. Repeat calls were made to Yashaswini who did not answer her phone. Kavita from ARDSI-DC who had counselled Josie over the years advised, 'Let it be Josie, let him go in dignity' and finally, in the August heat, Josie cremated her beloved Su.

In these two cases, the incongruities between medical category, institution and values are visible. Medical categorizations view organ donation as a transference, i.e., from one body into another, rather than a research enterprise or object of study. So Su's body, because of the dementia, was seen as an unsuitable donor and his gift of life was rejected. Bureaucratic bungling and institutional inefficiencies also left the Sood family unable to donate even when they chose to. If these are people's experiences, it comes as little surprise that rates of organ donation remain so low. What remains unanswered is the comparative speed of the process if the resources of an illegal black market economy were brought to bear. What if these organs were being sold rather than donated? Would the limitations of age and infirmity supersede the brute force of lucre? Would donation have been more successful as commodity? Would a free gift of life been more respected if it were not quite so philanthropically given? These are questions beyond the scope of this book but do require further investigation. In the interim, the failed attempts of these families at donation were painful endings to a highly emotional experience. As Josie said, 'I was devastated by the fact that his body could not be donated to science because that would have been [one of] his last wishes'.

Conclusion

The key elements of a Bollywood *masa:la:* have been used to structure this chapter. In place of plot logic, singular themes and gritty realities, there have multiple narratives, interruptions, numerous threads and fantastic stories. Yet even as the threads began to unravel for people with dementia, there was still space for relations and affections. The poetry, dance and exchanges I have described highlight that the deeper human intimacies are still very much present and people with dementia respond to them. On one level, it is unseemly that I even need to write such a research finding with regards to interactions between 'normal' people and people with dementia. Affections, respect and a willingness to listen should be humane and axiomatic to any given interaction. But as was also highlighted, humanity is not always in surplus in the difficult tasks of caring and dying. As people prepare for their loved one's death, a different set of interventions comes to bear on the dying process.

Families' emotional preparations for the death of their loved one were shaped by cultural scripts associated with dying and the political economy of dying and donation. As the issues faced by Josie and the Sood family with respect to organ donation illustrate, there is a new biopolitics transpiring on people's bodies, drawing on the old inequities of age and illness to script new pains of loss and hurt. Further research is required into this area in conjunction with an examination of the intersections of global economies, nationalism and bioethics in organ donation in India.

Finally, in caring for people with dementia and in preparing for and dealing with death, *sevā*, relationality and reciprocity have been explicitly explored in numerous contexts ranging from families' homes to the OPDs and institutions of government. But love has only been alluded to, even though it is implicit within the care-giving process, influencing relations, power-plays and attempts to secure better treatments and even cures. Love was in the sweetness of sugar, in the longing for home, partnerships forged and efforts to retain identity. Karamjit who showed off Nina's cross-stitch, big-hearted Shivbaksh who supplied Helen with her *biːɾiːs* and devoted Namita and her mother are all tales of love and loss. There are few happy endings in dementia care, but happily I found pockets of deep love and commitment. I now turn to documenting these intimacies in the final chapter.

CONCLUSION
'This is the Time for Romance'

WHEN I WAS GROWING UP in Delhi, typically schoolboys and girls would exchange a few misty cards and college students would grow flirtatious over their Pepsis® on Valentine's Day. By 2008, things had changed significantly and Cupid's arrow had struck the psyche of all classes. In the morning my maid wished me a happy Valentine's Day, a friend text messaged felicitations for 'a beautiful and romantic day' and more messages followed from various companies encouraging me to buy their products to find true love. A typical message read: 'WILL U MEET UR VALENTINE. Get valentine day forecast from Expert astrologer. Dial 55181, Rs 6.99 pr.mm'. When I mentioned these messages to a staff member at ARDSI, he was contemptuous:

> Do you know the price of a single red rose today is Rs 80?
> *How much is it normally?*
> About Rs 2 each. And there has been a guard put on the garden of the vice-chancellor at St. Stephen's [College] because all the students are coming and plucking the flowers! It is madness!

I was astonished at this commercialization of love. It is not that Delhi is a loveless city – indeed most of its parks are filled with couples behind suspiciously rustling foliage. But Delhi is more grasping and less melodic than cities such as Mumbai or Kolkata. For all its claims to 'modernization' and 'development', gender inequities, gender-based violence, poverty, class politics and conservative values are still *du jour* in Delhi. On Valentine's Day, television and radio stations covered stories of Hindu fundamentalist groups looting card shops and beating up couples. Within this context of money, sex and violence, love seemed too soft an emotion and too easily appropriated by the forces of capitalism and lust.

Not so, as I was to discover. One afternoon, as I sat with Josie in her hallway, a single overhead light glowing and the rest of the house in darkness, she said, 'This is the time for romance'. Outside the sky had gone a mossy, earthy green, the signs of an ominous storm to come. When the storm comes, the wind peels paint flecks from the walls, water seeps under the doors and time seems to stop. Josie says:

> This disease has made everything so much more. We're not like every other couple, husband here, wife there. He is totally dependent on me and I treasure every moment. It is such a joy to look after him because I know I've only got him for another few years. See, the sexual side of my life is gone. It's gone because of the disease and because of age. Our relationship has been transformed and he is now like my child. But I love to meet and talk to people. Especially to men – older men I prefer. Just to have a great conversation, for them to say, 'Hey, you're a great person to talk to'. I can't stand pity and all this *becharre* ('poor me') stuff. I say, 'Look, everyone has a job and this is my job and I am doing it. That's it'. But I treasure these moments, these flashes. He calls me 'lovely' and the other day, after months, when we were in church, he took my hand and said, 'You're so cute'. I felt like a young bride all over again.

To discover the love that existed between people with dementia and their spouses was one of the most joyous findings of my ethnographic journey. It was unexpected for there are few joyful finales with Alzheimer's disease. Death is inevitable and for many, this brings release and marks a huge life change after many years of caring. Perhaps because of the tragedies of the story and the intensity and intimacies of caring, carers and people with dementia shared a deep love. From Tandon who spent his days eternally hopeful and searching for a cure for Sheila to Nina who struggled to maintain Karamjit's function and identity, from Shivbaksh who cooked incessantly for Helen to the hungry oceanographer who yelled across his living room to his wife, 'Darling, what's for lunch?', there were stories of love and devotion.

Academia has not been rigorous about love. Love is taboo. Much has been written about affect, relationality, reciprocity, cohesion and exchange; about the substantive processes of love such as family planning, blood and kinship, childcare, eldercare, domesticity; and the commoditization of love in an era of late capitalism through sex work, transnational caregiving and reproductive tourism. Almost nothing has been written academically about the romance of love. Yet, it is one of the key lubricants of human relations, driving people to form kinship networks and connect with each other.

To write about love is to risk romanticizing one's work, the field and its players. But anthropology is a discipline that speaks most to falling in love.

One learns to love one's topic, to be passionate about it, to be immersed in a 'field', an alien space that the anthropologist endeavours to make familiar. Anthropology is much like migration – terrifying to begin with but eventually a site where a 'home' can be built. To be in love, anthropologically speaking, need neither preclude a critical gaze on our participants' lives nor the wider political context that shapes their identities and actions. Both views are necessary to capture the complexity of the topic and to do better justice to what we have been privy to. And so in this final chapter, as all the threads are woven together, I write first *of love* and then *with love*, of the analysis of the key themes that have defined this book.

'Any Sadness of Mine He Endeavoured to Make Sweet'

The couples in this study were of a generation that married young and usually through arrangements brokered by their families. Four couples had not even met their prospective spouses until the actual marriage itself. Helen and Shivbaksh were married off as children, when she was ten and he fifteen years old. The duties of work and childcare had governed most of their lives and many couples described long periods of separation – husbands who were stationed in military zones, out on the ocean, in tea gardens or at far-flung government posts, while wives lived elsewhere raising their children.

Throughout most of these couples' lives, love would have been akin to what Margaret Trawick (1990b) described in south Indian Tamil families. Love or *anpu*, according to Trawick, was articulated through living rather than speaking and encompassed numerous features such as *adakkam* (containment), *parakkam* (habit), *kodumai* (cruelty), *elimai* (simplicity) and *adimai* (servitude). Mothers were meant to be contained in their affections for their children and spouses restrained in the affections they showed each other. Too much love was believed to hurt both the giver and the receiver and threaten family unity. Love was seen to grow over time and included cruelty towards one's children with the intention of hardening them to the struggles of life and teaching them to appreciate the sweetness of success. Simplicity of living and service towards others, through processes such as preparing and serving food, were also aspects of *anpu*.

With retirement and illness, as the dementia progressed and institutional and social barriers hardened, couples found their relationships significantly changing. Some of the features of love as described by Trawick held true in my sample, but other aspects, such as containment and simplicity, did not. Distal forces, such as globalization, transnationalism and urbanization over time and immediate factors such as the nature of the illness and changes in family structure, contributed to these altered understandings of love.

While carers were contained in their displays of affection towards their loved one, they did not curtail themselves in describing their affections. Notions of simplicity were quickly displaced by the complexities of *sevā* and the details of carework. Days were spent focusing more and more on the minutiae of bodies and function. *Sevā* and duty increasingly came to the fore. Spouses tended to invoke the reciprocity of long years of marriage for their current caregiving:

> Whatever I can do, I do. He is my husband . . . as long as he is alive till then [it] is my duty. All these years he has kept me happy, so the least I can do is this (*Radha Menon, 62*).

> Now it doesn't matter to him how we keep him but in my heart it matters because I have always lived well with him. That's why we desire that he experience no difficulties because of us. We only want the best of the best for him (*Shafia Khan, 54*).

Family and wider social relations were also changed by dementia. People's lives tended to shrink in the public space that they occupied. There were fewer outings and lives eventually contracted to focus only onto beds and bathrooms. Adult children were often overseas, interstate, lived elsewhere in the city or were preoccupied with their own lives. Spouses were left alone to care and for many these were years of introspection and loneliness. Some people, such as Tandon, literally began to mobilize their solitude – through the physical spaces of their houses and outside walls – to keep visitors at bay.

The shifting of power dynamics and tighter disciplinary routines governing daily life also required carers to assume responsibility for tasks that were once beyond their purview. Women juggled finances, tax returns and administrative matters outside the home, while men had to focus on household chores and run an establishment. As their scope of responsibilities expanded, carers often found themselves experiencing an emotional distance from the rest of their extended family and friends who could not wholly empathize with their experiences. The combination of increasing emotional distance from family and friends, contracting of activities within the public sphere, notions of reciprocity and *sevā* and greater awareness of the chores the person with dementia used to perform, all strengthened the bonds between carers and people with dementia. Nina's remarks illustrate this dynamic:

We'll have our fiftieth anniversary this year. And we've had our ins and outs, seven year itches and all that. First it was husband-wife. You have to do this, I have to do this. You have your duty, I have my duty. You are together, be together. But now it is a comradeship, it is a friendship, it is as I would call it, love. It's not sex but love. Pure, simple love. I think that if a man loses his identity he is lost. What has he got left if I am not known as Nina Bhagat?

Women were more open about their feelings for their spouses than male carers. Six women explicitly mentioned how strongly they felt for their husbands and the love that they shared. For some, love was also tied to power and control because despite the difficulties of caring, they attained greater authority over their own and their husband's lives through such work. As Nina put it, 'Tomorrow if he is not there, the family will say, "Why are you doing this? Why are you doing that?" But now, nobody can question me'. Others, such as Sita Aggarwal who cared for her husband in her son's home, enjoyed little autonomy, bound as she was by the limitations of her husband's late-stage dementia and her dependence on her son for a roof over their heads.

Only two men in my sample were the primary carers for their wives – Shivbaksh and Govind Ballabh Tandon; the others shared this task with their daughters or daughters-in-law. For these two men, love was an emotion not readily admitted. Tandon said it was personal and Shivbaksh associated love with lust and passion, believing it to be something that occurred during one's youth. At eighty-seven, Shivbaksh believed that such amorous feelings were over for him and so when I bluntly asked him whether he loved Helen, he replied, 'What love? What is love? In old age there is no love. This is duty, this is obligation and there is no love between us'. He gave me this answer in early May 2008. By the end of June, Helen was dead and when I went for my final visit in August, I asked him again, 'Did you love Helen?' His answer was as follows: 'Love comes in old age. I cared for her, I did *sevā* for her, I did everything. Love was going to happen under these circumstances. Now she is gone and I am alone.'

'Now I am the Mother. Earlier she was the Mother'

> I always tell her, 'We were your babies, now you've become my baby. I don't have two daughters, now I have three daughters, you are my daughter' (Kumud Kaul).

Dementia also inversed the traditional parent-child dyad, with children caring for their parents, likening such work to the childcare their parents had provided them. Both Kumud and Nayantara, in separate interviews, stated that they felt that they were now mother to their mother, Mrs Hamdari. The same analogy held true for many other women caring for an ageing parent (but not for daughters-in-law who cared for in-laws with dementia). While understandings of *sevā* informed these relationships, the mother-child paradigm enhanced the love, power and intensity of this dynamic. Unlike the containment of the traditional mother-child bond, in these cases daughters showered affection on their mothers.

Love was displayed through gestures rather than speech. In the words of Deborah Hoffmann from the film *Complaints of a Dutiful Daughter* (1994), 'The content didn't matter; it was the feeling'. Children would stroke their mothers' hair, kiss their cheeks, apply makeup and ensure they were well presented. Watching TV together, lying down together and holding hands were instances of love and exchange. Just as food played a critical role in fostering love between spouses, feeding and eating also created feelings of love between parents and children. Kumud and Nayantara would often take their parents out to lunch at their local club:

> At least three to four times in a month, we make it a point to take them out. She feels very happy. Initially there is a lot of reluctance [laughs] and she'll go on saying, 'What shall I wear, I have no clothes'. And we sit at the dining table wherever we go; Nayantara sits with daddy and I sit with mummy or one of us sits [with the other], so both of us are there to look after them. Always, always.

Children's indulgence of their parents was underpinned by the knowledge that death was the end result. Restraining one's love was unnecessary because the person with dementia had already endured the hardships and sweetness of life. As Bhageshwari explained:

> The one thing that wears me down is that I know my mom is not going to survive for a very long time. Everyone has a dark spot in their lives, this is mine. I know she is not going to live for very long. It brings me down very badly. Everything else I can take in my stride. It's ok as long as I can see that smile on her face. It's not the pressure of doing [things] for her, it's not a pressure. As long as I see that she is feeling ok, it's fine. Some people find caring for parents a hindrance but for me, if she is around me, there is a sense of calm within me.

Key Themes

> Little events, ordinary things, smashed and reconstituted.
> Imbued with new meaning.
> Suddenly they become the bleached bones of a story.
>   – Arundhati Roy, *The God of Small Things* (1997: 32–33).

With illness and age, in an urban landscape, in a time of social and economic transformation and greater dialogue between India and the rest of the world, notions of love also shift. Previous adages of love as contained, habitual, simple, cruel and servile no longer apply. Love is linked to power and framed by age, illness and loss. Its manifestations are gendered and shaped by a history of reciprocity and exchange of bodily substance codes. Love is tragic and pleasurable, less spoken of and more an emotion that is displayed. Whether in the couples of this study, the parent-child relations, or in the young Delhi romantics on Valentine's Day, love is neither as contained nor as simple as it used to be.

Love, however, remained closely related to *sevā* and includes the range and depth of families' commitment and love for each other. *Sevā* is a culturally specific term that has resonated throughout this book. It is explicitly linked to power and discipline in everyday domesticities governing cooking, feeding and eating alongside other activities such as doctor shopping, the pursuit of an *ilāj* and bearing the costs associated with caring. *Sevā* flows across kin networks and not just between immediate relations. The elegance of *sevā* lies in its intricacies, in how it can hold people together, invoke reciprocity and shared memory, cultural ideas of love, duty and devotion, while still leaving space to explore the negativities of carework – the coercion, abuse and surveillance – that transpires within the home.

Sevā also feeds into the institutions of medicine, law and property, which in turn determine how care should be given and the incentives and admonishments associated with deviating from these standards. In this political economy of care the dialectic between the institutions of the state and cultural understandings such as *sevā* mutually reinforce the family's role in caring. Doctors' directives to relatives to care on delivering the dementia diagnosis and the polices' counsel to the aged to hold onto their property lest family members stop caring for them, are direct examples of how the state has firmly located the burden and costs of care entirely on the family.

There is also a historically shaped link between consumption and carers' identities. A 'good' carer is one who will spend money in search of a cure and leave no option untried in biomedicine, traditional and transcendental medicines. Doing *sevā* motivated families to endure dominant-subordinate relations in the clinic, incur expenses such as medicines and diapers, hire attendants and strive to give pleasures, large and small, to the person with dementia. The journeys that carers took to try and give their loved ones solace and comfort – Nina and Karamjit's trip to Europe for his stem cell treatment, Radha and Rajesh's journeys to Kerala, Lakshmi Kumari and her family's return to Pakistan – are such examples.

But corralling the costs of care within the domestic sphere leaves families vulnerable to mercenaries and stories such as Josie's and Su's resonate here. Their narrative reminds us that a family's search for help can have exorbitant monetary and emotional costs and highlights the need for policy makers and doctors to rethink seriously how care and treatment is conceived and delivered. In the world's largest democracy, disparities in healthcare delivery, access to services and treatment by health professionals are felt by greater numbers and are deeply saddening. The question of access, citizenship and rights repeats itself throughout this work, with no easy answers. The lack of follow up of medications for the person with dementia by doctors, ARDSI-DC's privileging of its relationships with its funders over the families, families' exploitation of their attendants, the vulnerability of older women in their homes and failed cases of organ donation, all point to a system in crisis where people are largely left to self-educate and fend for themselves. One may hope that with economic development and greater investment in the health sector this may change. But that more money will somehow translate into a better health system for people is questionable. The process will take too long. If past history is any indicator, then corruption, bureaucracy and bribery are likely to waylay some of these funds. However, there is always hope, and comfort may be taken from two small facts: (1) India has a thriving civil society and political freedom wherein critics and activists are vociferous; and (2) the Government is responsive to these voices and has taken steps towards caring for older people through additional funding of geriatric services, greater investment in professional training, increased funding of research for the aged care sector and the establishment of a National Institute of Ageing (Government of India 2007).

In terms of the overall health system, rather than focusing only on capital and investment, substantive changes also need to be argued from a rights-based perspective. Injections of funds will not necessarily change the attitudes and approach of providers to people. Class and gender hierarchies are deeply embedded in the social fabric and a Western individual centred approach to human rights and patient rights cannot be directly transplanted in India. Instead what is needed is a cultural shift that is joined both to the relative political freedoms that Indian citizens enjoy and to the notions of love and *sevā* that frame relations. Building on such cultural foundations need not necessitate a static view of culture. Far from stagnant and unchanging, Indian culture is dynamic, fluid and adaptable. The way forward is perhaps, as Kleinman (2007, 2008, 2009) advocates, greater integration of the medical humanities with biomedicine and a focus on the art as well as the technicalities of care. Caregiving is a moral practice, inextricably bound with being human, realizing another's suffering and one's own agency in alleviating or augmenting that suffering. It is too important a task to locate solely within families and to paid attendants. Care must be seen as crucial to the praxis of health professionals. It goes to the heart of medicine and is fundamental to the therapeutic relationship.

Last Words

So where to from here?

Ten months and ten days after I began, I finished. I got on a plane to return to Delhi from Kerala to fly away from India. I remember my body and hair smelling of coconuts. I had had the famous *Āyurvedic* massage in Kerala. Two women stripped me down to nothing and slathered me with oil. They touched my head, back, neck, shoulders, breasts, arms, stomach, buttocks, legs, feet and toes. They saw every part of me, implored me to relax, to be less 'tight', but I could not comply. By the end of my stay in India, there I was, stark naked, exposed and being touched. *Quid pro quo* anthropologist for all the bodies I had seen and touched here. People, who were naked and semi-clothed, dignified and maligned, their bodies old, enfeebled, young and vigorous. Yet I was unable to apply the matter-of-factness I applied to these bodies to my own.

Perhaps these will be my lessons. That the casualness with which we analyse and evaluate others, in anthropology and the clinic, does not apply to our own lives. That the rhetoric of care and 'expertise' belies an amorphous reality wherein there are few experts and learning by trial and error is commonplace. That love, power and *sevā* are more intense and complex processes than can be absorbed in the term 'care'. That in an era of globalization, money and transnationalism, the 'badness' of modern families that Cohen described (1998) is there but dissipating, the social ties that bound Lamb's (2000) Mangaldihi villagers endures but has thinned. That dialogue between India and abroad is occurring at all levels and the conversations are more ambiguous and less certain. I write my own farewell note to my grandmother, which is slipped into her coffin:

> *You are one of the most extraordinary and resilient people I have known in my life and I feel profound sorrow but also tremendous joy for your passing. Joy because your life has been defined by a great achievement that few can claim to have accomplished to the extent you have; you have birthed, raised and forged a truly transnational family. The bonds that you have created and invoked between us all, in health and through your illness, carry across oceans and across generations. Your life has taught us what it means to care and to care deeply. The intimacies and love that we share has made us all more human, more resilient and better people. So while I am so sad to lose you, I celebrate the legacy you leave and send you all my love as you are released from long years of suffering and reunited body, mind and soul in a better place. Grandpa will be waiting there for you.*

GLOSSARY

A:dmī:	Husband. Can also be a descendant of Adam; a human being; man; individual, person
A:ya:	Maid
Āyurveda	A type of Indian medicinal system (*āyus* means longevity; *veda* is knowledge)
Bahū	Daughter-in-law
Barsathi	A one-room or two-room habitation on the terrace of a building usually for renting purpose
Bechara	Poor thing; a creature to be pitied
Beta	Child; literally means son but is used to address both genders
Bha:bhi	Sister-in-law
Bhaiya:	Brother
Bhojan	Eating and giving food to others to eat
Bhūlnā	Memory loss; forgetfulness
Bi:ṛi:s	Unfiltered cigarettes
Buddhāpan	Old age
Būṛhā	Old people
Cha:y	Tea
Dādā	Paternal grandfather
Dādī	Paternal grandmother
Dal	Lentils
Dekh	See
Dekhānā:	To show
Dekhnā:	To see
Didi	Older sister
Dikhnā	To be seen
Doctor *sāhib*	Doctor sir
Gāyatrī-mantra	Highly revered mantra, based on a Vedic Sanskrit verse from the *Ṛgveda*
Ghar ka kha:na	Home cooking
Guru	Teacher, mentor and spiritual guide
Guṣṣa	Anger

Ḥakīm	Doctor in *Unani* medicine
Hāth-pair	Hands and feet; used to suggest the functionality of the body
Ilāj	'Cure' and 'to treat medically' in Hindi, Urdu, Persian, Arabic and Turkish
Jhāṛ-poṅćh	Conjuring, exorcizing; incantation, sorcery, hocus-pocus (particularly to cure a disease)
Kala jādū	Black magic
Kāmzori	Weakness
K͟hāmosh	Silence
Kurta:s	A kind of tunic
Masa:la:	Spices
Mātāji	A term of respect for a maternal figure
Nani-ma	Maternal grandmother
Pa:gaal	Mad
Parathas	Unleavened flatbreads made by pan-frying whole wheat flour. Often served hot and drizzled with ghee
Pra-ŋām	Blessing from an older person
Prasād	Food that is blessed from the temple
Rotis	Unleavened flatbreads made from wheat flour without oil (unlike *parathas* which are fried)
Sarkari	Government
Saṭhiyānā	'Gone sixtyish', to become senile
Sevā	Service, filial respect
Ṭhākur	Feudal lord or powerful land owner
Vaid	*Āyurvedic* doctor
Wallah	Suffix used to indicate a person involved in some kind of activity
Unani	Islamic medicinal systems with Greek roots
Zid	Stubbornness

REFERENCES

Aboderin, I. 2004. 'Modernisation and Ageing Theory Revisited: Current Explanations of Recent Developing World and Historical Western Shifts in Material Family Support for Older People', *Ageing and Society* 24(1): 29–50.
Administration on Aging. 2013. 'Profile of older Americans: 2011'. Washington DC.
Agarwal, B. 1998. 'Widows versus Daughters Or Widows as Daughters? Property, Land and Economic Security in Rural India', *Modern Asian Studies* 32(1): 1–48.
Ali, S. 2002. 'Collective and Elective Ethnicity: Caste among Urban Muslims in India', *Sociological Forum* 17(4): 593–620.
Alter, J. 2000. *Gandhi's Body: Sex, Diet, and the Politics of Nationalism*. Philadelphia: University of Pennsylvania Press.
_____. 2005. 'Introduction: The Politics of Culture and Medicine', in J.S. Alter (ed.), *Asian Medicine and Globalization*. Philadelphia: University of Pennsylvania Press, pp. 1–20.
The Alzheimer's and Related Disorders Society of India. 2006. http://www.mykerala.net/alzheimer/, accessed on 4 September 2007.
_____ 2010. 'The Dementia India Report: Prevalence, Impact, Costs and Services for Dementia'. New Delhi.
Alzheimer's Australia. 2007. 'Early Diagnosis of Dementia'. Canberra.
Alzheimer's Disease International. 2009. 'No Time to Lose!' http://www.alz.co.uk/adi/wad/wad2008.html, accessed on 5 March 2009.
Alzheimer's UK. 2013. 'Drug Treatments for Alzheimer's Disease'. http://www.alzheimers.org.uk/site/scripts/documents_info.php?documentID=147, accessed on 20 December 2013.
The American Psychiatric Association. 2000. 'Diagnostic Criteria from DSM-IV'. Washington DC.
_____ 2013. *Diagnostic and Statistical Manual of Mental Disorders, Fifth Edition. DSM 5*. Washington DC.
Angen, M. 2000. 'Evaluating Interpretive Inquiry: Reviewing the Validity Debate and Opening the Dialogue', *Qualitative Health Research* 10(3): 378–95.
Annerstedt, L. et al. 2000. 'Family Caregiving in Dementia: An Analysis of the Caregiver's Burden and the "Breaking-Point" when Home Care Becomes Inadequate', *Scandanavian Journal of Public Health* 28(1): 23–31.
Appadurai, A. 1981. 'Gastro-Politics in Hindu South Asia', *American Ethnologist* 8(3): 494–511.

_____ 1988. 'How to Make a National Cuisine: Cookbooks in Contemporary India', *Comparative Studies in Society and History* 30(1): 3–24.

_____ 1996. *Modernity at Large: Cultural Dimensions of Globalization*. Minneapolis: University of Minnesota Press.

Arlt, S. et al. 2008. 'Adherence to Medication in Patients with Dementia Predictors and Strategies for Improvement', *Drugs and Aging* 25(12): 1033–47.

Arnold, D. 1993. *Colonizing the Body: State Medicine and Epidemic Disease in Nineteenth-Century India*. Berkeley: University of California Press.

_____ 1996. 'The Rise of Western Medicine in India', *Lancet* 348(9034): 1075–78.

Askham, J. et al. 2007. 'Care at Home for People with Dementia: As in a Total institution?', *Ageing and Society* 27(1): 3–24.

Astin, J. et al. 1998. 'A Review of The Incorporation of Complementary and Alternative Medicine by Mainstream Physicians', *Archives of Internal Medicine* 158(21): 2303–10.

Australian Bureau of Statistics. 2013. 'Where and How do Australia's Older People Live? Reflecting a Nation: Stories from the 2011 Census', Catalogue 2071.0. Canberra.

Bala, P. 2007. *Medicine and Medical Policies in India: Social and Historical Perspectives*. Lanham: Lexington Books.

Baldassar, L., C.V. Baldock and R. Wilding. 2007. *Families Caring Across Borders: Migration, Ageing and Transnational Caregiving*. Basingstoke: Palgrave Macmillan.

Ballenger, J.F. 2006. 'The Biomedical Deconstruction of Senility and the Persistent Stigmatization of Old Age in the United States', in A. Leibing and L. Cohen (eds), *Thinking about Dementia: Culture, Loss, and the Anthropology of Senility*. New Brunswick: Rutgers University Press, pp. 106–120.

Banerjee, S. et al. 2003. 'Predictors of Institutionalisation in People with Dementia', *Journal of Neurology, Neurosurgery and Psychiatry* 74(9): 1315–16.

Banerji, D. 1978. 'Political Dimensions of Health and Health Services', *Economic and Political Weekly* 13(22): 924–28.

_____ 1981. 'The Place of Indigenous and Western Systems of Medicine in the Health Services of India', *Social Science and Medicine* 15A(2): 109–14.

Barnett, J.R. and R.A. Kearns. 1996. 'Shopping Around? Consumerism and the Use of Private Accident and Medical Clinics in Auckland, New Zealand', *Environment and Planning A* 28(6): 1053–75.

Bartlett, H. and W. Martin. 2002. 'Ethical Issues in Dementia Care Research', in H. Wilkinson (ed.), *The Perspectives of People with Dementia: Research Methods and Motivation*. London: Jessica Kingsley, pp. 47–62.

Bartlett, R. and D. O'Connor. 2007. 'From Personhood to Citizenship: Broadening the Lens for Dementia Practice and Research', *Journal of Aging Studies* 21(2): 107–18.

Basting, A.D. 2009. *Forget Memory: Creating Better Lives for People with Dementia*. Baltimore: Johns Hopkins University Press.

Bates, D.G. 1995. 'Scholarly Ways of Knowing: An Introduction', in D.G. Bates (ed.), *Knowledge and the Scholarly Medical Traditions*. Cambridge: Cambridge University Press, pp. 1–22.

Beard, R.L. and P.J. Fox. 2008. 'Resisting Social Disenfranchisement: Negotiating Collective Identities and Everyday Life with Memory Loss', *Social Science and Medicine* 66(7): 1509–20.

Bennett, E. 1999. 'Soft Truth: Ethics and Cancer in Northeast Thailand', *Anthropology and Medicine* 6(3): 395–404.

Berrios, G.E. and R. Porter. 1995. *A History of Clinical Psychiatry: The Origin and History of Psychiatric Disorders*. New York: New York University Press.

Beteille, A. 1997. 'Caste in Contemporary India', in C.J. Fuller (ed.), *Caste Today*. Delhi: Oxford University Press, pp. 150–79.

Bhat, A.K. and R. Dhruvarajan. 2001. 'Ageing in India: Drifting Intergenerational Relations, Challenges and Options', *Ageing and Society* 21(5): 621–40.

Bhatia, B.M. 1967. *Famines in India: A Study in Some Aspects of the Economic History of India, 1860-1965*, 2nd edn. Bombay: Asia Publishing House.

Biehl, J. 2004. 'Life of the Mind: The Interface of Psychopharmaceuticals, Domestic Economies, and Social Abandonment', *American Ethnologist* 31(4): 475–96.

Biswas, P. and A. Biswas. 2007. 'Setting Standards for Proactive Pharmacovigilance in India: The Way Forward', *Indian Journal of Pharmacology* 39(3): 124–28.

Biswas, S. 2013. 'Do India's "Fast Track" Courts Work?' BBC News India. http://www.bbc.co.uk/news/world-asia-india-20944633, accessed on 19 December 2013.

Bourdieu, P. 1990. *The Logic of Practice*. Stanford: Stanford University Press.

Bradburd, D. and W.R. Jankowiak. 2003. 'Drugs, Desire and European Economic Expansion', in W.R. Jankowiak and D. Bradburd (eds), *Drugs, Labor and Colonial Expansion*. Tucson: University of Arizona Press, pp. 3–29.

Braekhus, A., et al. 1998. 'Social and Depressive Stress Suffered by Spouses of Patients with Mild Dementia', *Scandanavian Journal of Primary Health Care* 16(4): 242–46.

Breckenridge, C.A. 1995. *Consuming Modernity: Public Culture in a South Asian World*. Minneapolis: University of Minnesota Press.

Briggs, K. et al. 2003. 'Accomplishing Care at Home for People with Dementia: Using Observational Methodology', *Qualitative Health Research* 13(2): 268–80.

Brijnath, B. 2008. 'The Legislative and Political Contexts Surrounding Dementia Care in India', *Ageing and Society* 28(7): 913–34.

———— 2009. 'Familial Bonds and Boarding Passes: Understanding Caregiving in a Transnational Context', *Identities – Global Studies in Culture and Power* 16(1): 83–101.

———— 2011a. 'Screening for Dementia: Fluidity and the MMSE in India', *Transcultural Psychiatry* 48(5): 604–23.

———— 2011b. 'Use of the MMSE to Screen for Dementia in Delhi', *Dementia* 10(4): 625–35.

Brijnath, B. and L. Manderson. 2008. 'Discipline in Chaos: Foucault, Dementia and Aging in India', *Culture Medicine and Psychiatry* 32(4): 607–26.

———— 2011. 'Appropriation and Dementia in India', *Culture, Medicine and Psychiatry* 35(4): 501–18.

Brodaty, H. 2005. *Six Reasons Why Early Diagnosis of Dementia Does Not Occur and Ten Reasons Why It Should*. Canberra: Alzheimer's Australia.

Brodaty, H. and A. Green. 2002. 'Who Cares for the Carer? The Often Forgotten Patient', *Australian Family Physician* 31(9): 833–36.

Brooker, D. 2007. *Person Centred Dementia Care: Making Services Better*. London: Jessica Kingsley.
Bryden, C. 2005. *Dancing with Dementia: My Story of Living Positively with Dementia*. London: Jessica Kingsley.
Butalia, U. 2002. 'An Archive with a Difference: Partition Letters', in S. Kaul (ed.), *The Partitions of Memory: The Afterlife of the Division of India*. Bloomington: Indiana University Press, pp. 208–41.
Cadène, P. 2000. 'Delhi's Place in India's Urban Structure', in V. Dupont, E. Tarlo and D. Vidal (eds), *Delhi: Urban Space and Human Destinies*. New Delhi: Manohar Publishers and Distributors, pp. 241–49.
Cammann, S. 1969. 'Islamic and Indian Magic Squares. Part I', *History of Religions* 8(3): 181–209.
Carpenter, H. et al. 1996. 'The Politics of Drug Distribution in Bohol, the Philippines', *Asian Studies Review* 20(1): 35–52.
Census of India. 2011. *Census Info India Dashboard*. New Delhi: Office of the Registrar General and Census Commissioner.
Chacko, E. 2003. 'Culture and Therapy: Complementary Strategies for the Treatment of Type-2 Diabetes in an Urban Setting in Kerala, India', *Social Science and Medicine* 56(5): 1087–98.
Chatterjee, P. 1990. 'The Nationalist Resolution of the Women's Question', in K. Sangari and S. Vaid (eds), *Recasting Women: Essays in Indian Colonial History*. New Brunswick: Rutgers University Press, pp. 233–53.
Chattopadhyay, S. 2002. '"Goods, Chattels and Sundry Items": Constructing 19th-Century Anglo-Indian Domestic Life', *Journal of Material Culture* 7(3): 243–71.
Chaudhary, N. and P. Bhargava. 2006. 'Mamta: The Transformation of Meaning in Everyday Usage', *Contributions to Indian Sociology* 40(3): 343–73.
Chen, M. and J. Dreze. 1995. 'Recent Research on Widows in India: Workshop and Conference Report', *Economic and Political Weekly* 30(39): 2435–50.
Cohen, L. 1998. *No Aging in India: Alzheimer's, The Bad Family, and Other Modern Things*. Berkeley: University of California Press.
_____ 2001. 'The Other Kidney: Biopolitics Beyond Recognition', *Body and Society* 7(2–3): 9–29.
_____ 2006. 'Introduction: Thinking about Dementia', in A. Leibing and L. Cohen (eds), *Thinking about Dementia: Culture, Loss, and the Anthropology of Senility*. New Brunswick: Rutgers University Press, pp. 1–19.
Col, N., J.E. Fanale and P. Kronholm. 1990. 'The Role of Medication Noncompliance and Adverse Drug-Reactions in Hospitalisations of the Elderly', *Archives of Internal Medicine* 150(4): 841–45.
Coleman, L. 2009. 'Being Alone Together: From Solidarity to Solitude in Urban Anthropology', *Anthropological Quarterly* 82(3): 755–78.
Connell, R.W. 1995. *Masculinities*. St. Leonards: Allen and Unwin.
Cooney, C., R. Howard and B. Lawlor. 2006. 'Abuse of Vulnerable People with Dementia by Their Carers: Can We Identify Those Most at Risk?', *International Journal of Geriatric Psychiatry* 21(6): 564–71.

Copeman, J. 2004. '"Blood Will Have Blood": A Study in Indian Political Ritual', *Social Analysis* 48(3): 126–48.
_____ 2006. 'Cadaver Donation as Ascetic Practice in India', *Social Analysis* 50(1): 103–26.
_____ 2009. 'Gathering Points: Blood Donation and the Scenography of "National Integration" in India', *Body and Society* 15(2): 71–99.
Corner, L. and J. Bond. 2004. 'Being at Risk of Dementia: Fears and Anxieties of Older Adults', *Journal of Aging Studies* 18(2): 143–55.
_____ 2006. 'The Impact of the Label of Mild Cognitive Impairment on the Individual's Sense of Self', *Philosophy, Psychiatry, and Psychology* 13(1): 3–12.
Crocker, J., B. Major and C. Steele. 1998. 'Social Stigma', in D. Gilbert, S.T. Fiske and G. Lindzey (eds), *The Handbook of Social Psychology*, 4th edn. New York: McGraw-Hill, pp. 504–53.
Csordas, T.J. 1990. 'Embodiment as a Paradigm for Anthropology', *Ethos* 18(1): 5–47.
Currie, B. 2000. *The Politics of Hunger in India: A Study of Democracy, Governance, and Kalahandi's Poverty*. New York: Macmillan Press.
Czymoniewicz-Klippel, M., B. Brijnath and B. Crockett. 2010. 'Ethics and the Promotion of Inclusiveness within Qualitative Research: Case Examples from Asia and the Pacific', *Qualitative Inquiry* 16(5): 332–41.
Dalal, A.K. 2000. 'Living with a Chronic Disease: Healing and Psychological Adjustment in Indian Society', *Psychology and Developing Societies* 12(1): 67–82.
Dalrymple, W. 1994. *City of Djinns: A Year in Delhi*. London: Flamingo.
Das, G. 2001. *India Unbound*. New York: A.A. Knopf.
Das, J. and J.S. Hammer. 2004. *Strained Mercy: The Quality of Medical Care in Delhi*. New Delhi: World Bank.
Das, V. 1976. 'The Uses of Liminality: Society and Cosmos in Hinduism', *Contributions to Indian Sociology* 10(2): 245–63.
_____ 1988. 'Femininity and Orientation to the Body', in K. Chanana (ed.), *Socialisation, Education and Women: Explorations in Gender Identity*. New Delhi: Orient Longman, pp. 193–207.
_____ 1998. 'Forms of Community in India: Solidarity, Crisis, and Representation', *XIV World Congress of Sociology*, Montreal: International Sociological Association.
_____ 2003. 'Technologies of Self: Poverty and Health in an Urban Setting', in R. Vasudevan et al. (eds), *Sarai Reader 2003: Shaping Technologies*. New Delhi: Sarai, pp. 95–102.
Das, V. and R. Addlakha. 2001. 'Disability and Domestic Citizenship: Voice, Gender, and the Making of the Subject', *Public Culture* 13(3): 511–32.
Das, V. and R.K. Das. 2006. 'Urban Health and Pharmaceutical Consumption in Delhi, India', *Journal of Biosocial Science* 38(1): 69–82.
Davies, B. et al. 2004. 'The Ambivalent Practices of Reflexivity', *Qualitative Inquiry* 10(3): 360–89.
Davis, D.H.J. 2004. 'Dementia: Sociological and Philosophical Constructions', *Social Science and Medicine* 58(2): 369–78.
Del Vecchio Good, M.J. et al. 1994. 'Oncology and Narrative Time', *Social Science and Medicine* 38(6): 855–62.

Deleuze, G. 1998. *Essays Critical and Clinical*. Minneapolis: University of Minnesota Press.
Delhi Police Senior Citizen's Cell. 2008. *Senior Citizen's Safety is Our Concern*. New Delhi.
Department of AYUSH. 2012. 'Summary of All-India AYUSH Infrastructure Facilities'. http://indianmedicine.nic.in/writereaddata/linkimages/5652579803-0I.pdf, accessed on 16 December 2013.
Deshpande, S. 1998. 'After Culture: Renewed Agendas for the Political Economy of India', *Cultural Dynamics* 10(2): 147–69.
Deshpande, S.G. and R. Tiwari. 1997. 'Self Medication: A Growing Concern', *Indian Journal of Medical Sciences* 51(3): 93–96.
Desjarlais, R. 1997. *Shelter Blues: Sanity and Selfhood among the Homeless*. Philadelphia: University of Pennsylvania Press.
Dewing, J. 2007. 'Participatory Research: A Method for Process Consent with Persons who have Dementia', *Dementia* 6(1): 11–25.
Dharmalingam, A. 1994. 'Old Age Support: Expectations and Experiences in a South Indian Village', *Population Studies* 48(1): 5–19.
Dias, A. et al. 2004. 'The Impact Associated with Caring for a Person with Dementia: A Report from the 10/66 Dementia Research Group's Indian Network', *International Journal of Geriatric Psychiatry* 19(2): 182–84.
Dossa, P. 2006. 'Disability, Marginality and the Nation-State – Negotiating Social Markers of Difference: Fahimeh's Story', *Disability and Society* 21(4): 345–58.
Douglas, M. 1966. *Purity and Danger: An Analysis of Concept of Pollution and Taboo*. London: Routledge.
Drèze, J. and A. Sen. 1989. *Hunger and Public Action*. Oxford: Oxford University Press.
———— 1990. *The Political Economy of Hunger*. Oxford: Oxford University Press.
Drèze, J., A. Sen and A. Hussain. 1995. *The Political Economy of Hunger: Selected Essays*. Oxford: Oxford University Press.
Dube, L. 1988. 'Socialisation of Hindu girls in Patrilineal India', in K. Chanana (ed.), *Socialisation, Education and Women: Explorations in Gender Identity*. New Delhi: Orient Longman, pp. 166–92.
Dumit, J. 2004. *Picturing Personhood: Brain Scans and Biomedical Identity*. Princeton: Princeton University Press.
Dumont, L. 1980. *Homo Hierarchicus: The Caste System and Its Implications*. Chicago: University of Chicago Press.
Dupont, V. 2000. 'Spatial and Demographic Growth of Delhi', in V. Dupont, E. Tarlo and D. Vidal (eds), *Delhi: Urban Space and Human Destinies*. New Delhi: Manohar Publishers and Distributors, pp. 229–39.
Eaton, L. 2002. 'Adverse Reactions to Drugs Increase', *British Medical Journal* 324(7328): 8.
Ecks, S. 2005. 'Pharmaceutical Citizenship: Antidepressant Marketing and the Promise of Demarginalization in India', *Anthropology and Medicine* 12(3): 239–54.

Emmatty, L.M., R.S. Bhatti and M.T. Mukalel. 2006. 'The Experience of Burden in India: A Study of Dementia Caregivers', *Dementia* 5(2): 223–32.
Farmer, P. 2003. *Pathologies of Power: Health, Human Rights, and the New War on the Poor*. Berkeley: University of California Press.
Farquhar, J. 2002. *Appetites: Food and Sex in Postsocialist China*. Durham: Duke University Press.
Fathers, M. 1999. 'Plight of the Living Dead', *TIME Asia*, 19 July. http://www.time.com/time/asia/asia/magazine/1999/990719/souls1.html, accessed on 20 December 2013.
Federal Interagency Forum on Aging-Related Statistics. 2012.
Older Americans 2012: Key Indicators of Well- Being. Washington DC.
Fernandes, L. 2006. *India's New Middle Class: Democratic Politics in an Era of Economic Reform*. Minneapolis: University of Minnesota Press.
Ferri, C.P. et al. 2005. 'Global Prevalence of Dementia: A Delphi Consensus Study', *Lancet* 366(9503): 2112–17.
Finkler, K. 1994. 'Sacred Healing and Biomedicine Compared', *Medical Anthropology Quarterly* 8(2): 178–97.
Fitzsimons, A. 2002. 'Masculinity at Work', in A. Fitzsimons (ed.), *Gender as a Verb: Gender Segregation at Work*. Aldershot: Ashgate, pp. 95–129.
Folstein, M.F., S.E. Folstein and P.R. McHugh. 1975. '"Mini-Mental State". A Practical Method for Grading the Cognitive State of Patients for the Clinician', *Journal of Psychiatric Research* 12(3): 189–98.
Foner, N. 1994. *The Caregiving Dilemma: Work in an American Nursing Home*. Berkeley: University of California Press.
Fontana, A. and R.W. Smith. 1989. 'Alzheimer's Disease Victims: The "Unbecoming" of Self and the Normalization of Competence', *Sociological Perspectives* 32(1): 35–46.
Foucault, M. 1975. *The Birth of the Clinic: An Archaeology of Medical Perception*. New York: Vintage Books.
_____ 1975, 2003. *Abnormal: Lectures at the Collège de France, 1974–1975*. London: Verso.
Foucault, M. and C. Gordon. 1980. *Power/Knowledge: Selected Interviews and Other Writings, 1972-1977*. Brighton: Harvester Press.
Foucault, M. and A. Sheridan. 1977. *Discipline and Punish: The Birth of the Prison*. London: Allen Lane.
Freidson, E. 1970. *Profession of Medicine: A Study of the Sociology of Applied Knowledge*. Chicago: University Of Chicago Press.
Fuller, C.J. 1996. 'Introduction', in C.J. Fuller (ed.), *Caste Today*. Delhi: Oxford University Press, pp. 1–31.
Gammeltoft, T.M. 2008. 'Childhood Disability and Parental Moral Responsibility in Northern Vietnam: Towards Ethnographies of Intercorporeality', *Journal of the Royal Anthropological Institute* 14(4): 825–42.
Ganti, T. 2004. *Bollywood: A Guidebook to Popular Hindi Cinema*. New York: Routledge.
Gardner, K. 1993. 'Mullahs, Migrants, Miracles: Travel and Transformation in Sylhet', *Contributions to Indian Sociology* 27(2): 213–35.

Ghavamzadeh, A. and B. Bahar. 1997. 'Communication with the Cancer Patient in Iran', *Annals of the New York Academy of Sciences* 809: 261–65.
Gikonyo, C. et al. 2008. 'Taking Social Relationships Seriously: Lessons Learned from the Informed Consent Practices of a Vaccine Trial on the Kenyan Coast', *Social Science and Medicine* 67(5): 708–20.
Gilman, S.L. 1996. *Seeing the Insane*. Lincoln: University of Nebraska Press.
Goel, D.S. et al. 2004. 'Mental Health 2003: The Indian Scene', in S.P. Agarwal (ed.), *Mental Health: An Indian Perspective 1946-2003*. New Delhi: Ministry of Health and Family Services, pp. 3–24.
Goffman, E. 1959. Reprinted 1990. *The Presentation of Self in Everyday Life*. London: Penguin Books.
_____ 1961. *Asylums: Essays on the Social Situation of Mental Patients and Other Inmates*. Garden City: Anchor Books.
_____ 1963, 1986. *Stigma: Notes on the Management of Spoiled Identity*. New York: Simon and Schuster.
Good, B.J. 1994. *Medicine, Rationality, and Experience: An Anthropological Perspective*. Cambridge: Cambridge University Press.
Goodman, L.E. 2009. 'al-Razi', in P. Bearman et al. (eds), *Encyclopedia of Islam*, 2nd edn. Brill Online. http://www.brillonline.nl/subscriber/entry?entry=islam_SIM-6267, accessed on 28 June 2013.
Gopalan, L. 2002. *Cinema of Interruptions: Action Genres in Contemporary Indian Cinema*. London: British Film Institute.
Gould, H. 1965. 'Modern Medicine and Folk Cognition in Rural India', *Human Organization* 24(3): 201–08.
Government of India. 2007. '11th Five Year Plan (2007-2011)'. New Delhi.
_____ 2012. '12th Five Year Plan (2012–2017)'. New Delhi.
_____ 2013. 'Press Notes on Poverty Estimates, 2011–2012'. New Delhi.
_____ 2006. 'Task Force for Planning on Human Resources in Health Sector'. New Delhi.
Government of National Capital Territory of Delhi. 2006. 'Morbidity, Health Care and Condition of Aged Persons in Delhi'. New Delhi.
Granado, S. et al. 2011. 'Appropriating "Malaria": Local Responses to Malaria Treatment and Prevention in Abidjan, Côte d'Ivoire', *Medical Anthropology* 30(1): 102–21.
Grbich, C. 2007. *Qualitative Data Analysis: An Introduction*. London: SAGE.
Greenhalgh, T. 1987. 'Drug Prescription and Self-Medication in India: An Exploratory Survey', *Social Science and Medicine* 25(3): 307–18.
Guillemin, M. and L. Gillam. 2004. 'Ethics, Reflexivity, and "Ethically Important Moments" in Research', *Qualitative Inquiry* 10(2): 261–80.
Gupta, C. 2002. *Sexuality, Obscenity, Community: Women, Muslims, and the Hindu Public in Colonial India*. New York: Palgrave.
Gururaj, G., N. Girish and M.K. Issac. 2005. *Mental, Neurological and Substance Abuse Disorders: Strategies Towards a Systems Approach*. New Delhi: National Commission on Macroeconomics and Health.
Hage, G. 2009. 'Hating Israel in the Field: On Ethnography and Political Emotions', *Anthropological Theory* 9(1), 59–79.

Hagihara, A. et al. 2005. 'A Signal Detection Approach to Patient-Doctor Communication and Doctor-Shopping Behaviour Among Japanese Patients', *Journal of Evaluation in Clinical Practice* 11(6): 556–67.

Hahn, H.P. 2004. 'Global Goods and the Process of Appropriation', in P. Probst and G. Spittler (eds), *Between Resistance and Expansion: Explorations of Local Vitality in Africa*. Munster: Lit Verlag, pp. 213–31.

Hall, A.J. et al. 2008. 'Patterns of Abuse among Unintentional Pharmaceutical Overdose Fatalities', *Journal of the American Medical Association* 300(22): 2613–20.

Haque, M.M., and K. Kusakabe. 2005. 'Retrenched Men Workers in Bangladesh: A Crisis of Masculinities?', *Gender, Technology and Development* 9(2): 185–208.

Harrison, M. 1994. *Public Health in British India: Anglo-Indian Preventive Medicine, 1859-1914*. Cambridge: Cambridge University Press.

Heath, I. 2003. 'A Wolf in Sheep's Clothing: A Critical Look at the Ethics of Drug Taking', *British Medical Journal* 327(7419): 856–58.

Hebert, R. et al. 2001. 'Factors Associated with Long-term Institutionalization of Older People with Dementia: Data from the Canadian Study of Health and Aging', *The Journal of Gerontology* 56A(11): M693–99.

Hellstrom, I. et al. 2007. 'Ethical and Methodological Issues in Interviewing Persons with Dementia', *Nursing Ethics* 14(5): 608–19.

Herzfeld, M. 1987. *Anthropology Through the Looking-Glass: Critical Ethnography in the Margins of Europe*. Cambridge: Cambridge University Press.

Hibberd, P. et al. 2009. 'Using Photographs and Narratives to Contextualise and Map the Experience of Caring for a Person with Dementia', *Journal of Nursing and Healthcare of Chronic Illness* 1(3): 215–28.

Hochschild, A. 1989. *The Second Shift: Working Parents and the Revolution at Home*. New York: Viking.

——— 2000. 'Global Care Chains and Emotional Surplus Value', in W. Hutton and A. Giddens (eds), *On the Edge: Living with Global Capitalism*. London: Jonathan Cape, pp. 15–30.

——— 2003. *The Managed Heart: Commercialization of Human Feeling*, 20th anniversary edn. Berkeley: University of California Press.

Holmes, E.R., and L.D. Holmes. 1995. *Other Cultures, Elder Years*, 2nd edn. Thousand Oaks: SAGE.

Holtzman, J.D. 2006. 'Food and Memory', *Annual Review of Anthropology* 35(1): 361–78.

Hux, M.J. et al. 1998. 'Relation between Severity of Alzheimer's Disease and Costs of Caring', *Canadian Medical Association Journal* 159(5): 457–65.

Ikels, C. 2002. 'Constructing and Deconstructing the Self: Dementia in China', *Journal of Cross Cultural Gerontology* 17(3): 233–51.

Isaksen, L.W. 2002. 'Toward a Sociology of (Gendered) Disgust: Images of Bodily Decay and the Social Organization of Care Work', *Journal of Family Issues* 23(7): 791–811.

Iype, T. et al. 2006. 'Usefulness of the Rowland Universal Dementia Assessment Scale in South India', *Journal of Neurology Neurosurgery and Psychiatry* 77(4): 513–14.

Jackson, C. 1999. 'Men's Work, Masculinities and Gender Divisions of Labour', *Journal of Development Studies* 36(1): 89–108.
Jackson, M. 1989. *Paths Toward a Clearing: Radical Empiricism and Ethnographic Inquiry*. Bloomington: Indiana University Press.
Jain, S. and S. Jadhav. 2008. 'A Cultural Critique of Community Psychiatry in India', *International Journal of Health Services* 38(3): 561–84.
Jamuna, D. 2003. 'Issues of Elder Care and Elder Abuse in the Indian Context', *Journal of Aging and Social Policy* 15(2/3): 125–42.
Jeffery, P. and R. Jeffery. 2008. '"Money Itself Discriminates": Obstetric Emergencies in the Time of Liberalisation', *Contributions to Indian Sociology* 42(1): 59–91.
Jeffery, R. 1988. *The Politics of Health in India*. Berkeley: University of California Press.
Johnston, J.M. et al. 2006. 'Non-Attendance and Effective Equity of Access at Four Public Specialist Outpatient Centers in Hong Kong', *Social Science and Medicine* 62(10): 2551–64.
Johnston, R.K. and T. Mann. 2000. 'Barriers to Antiretroviral Medication Adherence in HIV-Infected Women', *AIDS Care: Psychological and Socio-medical Aspects of AIDS/HIV* 12(4): 377–86.
Jones, E.E. 1984. *Social Stigma: The Psychology of Marked Relationships*. New York: W.H. Freeman.
Kakar, S. 1988. 'Feminine Identity in India', in R. Ghadially (ed.), *Women in Indian Society*. New Delhi: SAGE, pp. 44–68.
_____ 1990. *Intimate Relations: Exploring Indian Sexuality*. Chicago: University of Chicago Press.
_____ 1991. *The Analyst and the Mystic: Psychoanalytic Reflections on Religion and Mysticism*. Chicago: University of Chicago Press.
Kamat, V.R., and M. Nichter. 1997. 'Monitoring Product Movement: An Ethnographic Study of Pharmaceutical Sales Representatives in Bombay, India', in S. Bennett, B. McPake and A. Mills (eds), *Private Health Providers in Developing Countries: Serving the Public Interest?*. London: Zed Books, pp. 124–40.
_____ 1998. 'Pharmacies, Self-Medication and Pharmaceutical Marketing in Bombay, India', *Social Science and Medicine* 47(6): 779–94.
Kane, P.V. 1930, 1962. *History of Dharmasastra, 1962*, translated by P.V. Kane. Poona: Bhandarkar Oriental Research Institute.
Karner, T.X. 1998. 'Professional Caring: Homecare Workers as Fictive Kin', *Journal of Aging Studies* 12(1): 69–82.
Kaufert, J. 1999. 'Cultural Mediation in Cancer Diagnosis and End Of Life Decision-Making: The Experience of Aboriginal Patients in Canada', *Anthropology and Medicine* 6(3): 405–21.
Kaufman, S. 2006. 'Dementia-Near-Death and "Life Itself"', in A. Leibing and L. Cohen (eds), *Thinking about Dementia: Culture, Loss, and the Anthropology of Senility*. New Brunswick: Rutgers University Press, pp. 23–42.
Khan, S. 2006. 'Systems of Medicine and Nationalist Discourse in India: Towards "New Horizons" in Medical Anthropology and History', *Social Science and Medicine* 62(11): 2786–97.

Khare, R.S. 1976. *Culture and Reality: Essays on the Hindu System of Managing Foods*. Simla: Indian Institute of Advanced Study.
———— 1996. 'Dava, Daktar, and Dua: Anthropology of Practiced Medicine in India', *Social Science and Medicine* 43(5): 837–48.
———— 1998. 'The Issue of "Right to Food" among the Hindus: Notes and Comments', *Contributions to Indian Sociology* 32(2): 253–78.
Khare, R.S. and M.S. Rao. 1986. *Aspects in South Asian Food Systems: Food, Society, and Culture*. Durham: Carolina Academic Press.
Kirmayer, L.J. and A. Young. 1998. 'Culture and Somatization: Clinical, Epidemiological, and Ethnographic Perspectives', *Psychosomatic Medicine* 60(4): 420–30.
Kitwood, T. 1997. *Dementia Reconsidered: The Person Comes First*. Buckingham: Open University Press.
Kitwood, T. and K. Bredin. 1992. 'Towards a Theory of Dementia Care: Personhood and Well-Being', *Ageing and Society* 12(3): 269–87.
Kleinman, A. 1980. *Patients and Healers in the Context of Culture: An Exploration of the Borderland between Anthropology, Medicine and Psychiatry*. Berkeley: University of California Press.
———— 1999. 'Experience and its Moral Modes: Culture, Human Conditions, and Disorder', in G. B. Peterson (ed.), *The Tanner Lectures on Human Values*. Salt Lake City: University of Utah Press, pp. 357–420.
———— 2006. *What Really Matters: Living a Moral Life Amidst Uncertainty and Danger*. New York: Oxford University Press.
———— 2007. *Today's Biomedicine and Caregiving: Are they Incompatible to the Point of Divorce?* Paper presented at the als Cleveringa hoogleraar, Leiden: Universiteit Leiden.
———— 2008. 'Catastrophe and Caregiving: The Failure of Medicine as an Art', *Lancet* 371(9606): 22–23.
———— 2009. 'Caregiving: The Odyssey of Becoming More Human', *Lancet* 373(9660): 292–93.
Kleinman, A., V. Das and M. Lock. 1997. *Social Suffering*. Berkeley: University of California Press.
Kleinman, A. and E. Fitz-Henry. 2007. 'Experiential Basis of Subjectivity', in J.G. Biehl, B.J. Good and A. Kleinman (eds), *Subjectivity: Ethnographic Investigations*. Berkeley: University of California Press, pp. 52–65.
Kleinman, A. and B.J. Good. 1985. *Culture and Depression: Studies in the Anthropology and Cross-Cultural Psychiatry of Affect and Disorder*. Berkeley: University of California Press.
Kleinman, A. and J. Kleinman. 1991. 'Suffering and its Professional Transformation: Toward an Ethnography of Interpersonal Experience', *Culture Medicine and Psychiatry* 15(3): 275–301.
Kleinman, A. and D. Seeman. 1999. 'The Politics of Moral Practice in Psychotherapy and Religious Healing', in V. Das, D. Gupta and P. Uberoi (eds), *Tradition, Pluralism and Identity: In Honour of T.N. Madan*. New Delhi: SAGE Publications, pp. 95–110.
Knopman, D.S. et al. 2001. 'Practice Parameter: Diagnosis of Dementia (An Evidence-Based Review). Report of the Quality Standards Subcommittee of the American Academy of Neurology', *Neurology* 56(9): 1143–53.

Kontos, P.C. 2006. 'Embodied Selfhood: An Ethnographic Exploration of Alzheimer's Disease', in A. Leibing and L. Cohen (eds), *Thinking about Dementia: Culture, Loss, and the Anthropology of Senility*. New Brunswick: Rutgers University Press, pp. 195–217.

Kontos, P.C. and G. Naglie. 2007. 'Expressions of Personhood in Alzheimer's Disease: An Evaluation of Research-based Theatre as a Pedagogical Tool', *Qualitative Health Research* 17(6): 799–811.

Kumar, N. 1992. *Friends, Brothers, and Informants: Fieldwork Memoirs of Banaras*. Berkeley: University of California Press. http://ark.cdlib.org/ark:/13030/ft6x0nb4g3/, UC Press E-books Collection: 1982-2004, accessed on 26 August 2009.

Kumar, S.J. 1996. 'The Aged and Aged Disabled: The Indian Scene', *International Review of Modern Sociology* 26(1): 81–90.

Lal, N. 2008. 'Huge Case Backlog Clogs India's Courts', Asia Times Online. http://www.atimes.com/atimes/South_Asia/JF28Df02.html, accessed on 28 June 2008.

Lamb, S. 2000. *White Saris and Sweet Mangoes: Aging, Gender, and Body in North India*. Berkeley: University of California Press.

_____ 2005. 'Cultural and Moral Values Surrounding Care and (In)Dependence in Late Life: Reflections from India in an Era of Global Modernity', *Care Management Journals* 6(2): 80–89.

_____ 2009. *Aging and the Indian Diaspora: Cosmopolitan Families in India and Abroad*. Bloomington: Indiana University Press.

Lan, P.C. 2002. 'Subcontracting Filial Piety: Elder Care in Ethnic Chinese Immigrant Families in California', *Journal of Family Issues* 23(7): 812–35.

Lang, L.T. 1990. 'Aspects of the Cambodian Death and Dying Process', in J.K. Parry (ed.), *Social Work Practice with the Terminally Ill: A Transcultural Perspective*. Springfield: C.C. Thomas, pp. 205–11.

Langford, J. 1999. 'Medical Mimesis: Healing Signs of a Cosmopolitan "Quack"', *American Ethnologist* 26(1): 24–46.

_____ 2002. *Fluent Bodies: Ayurvedic Remedies for Postcolonial Imbalance*. Durham: Duke University Press.

_____ 2003. 'Traces of Folk Medicine in Jaunpur', *Cultural Anthropology* 18(3): 271–303.

Lau, L.J. 2006. 'The New Indian Woman: Who is She, and What is "New" about Her?', *Women's Studies International Forum* 29(2): 159–71.

The Laws of Manu. c. 500 BC. Trans. G. Bèuhler. 1964. Delhi: Motilal Banarsidas.

Lawton, J. 1998. 'Contemporary Hospice Care: The Sequestration of the Unbounded Body and "Dirty Dying"', *Sociology of Health and Illness* 20(2): 121–43.

Lee-Treweek, G. 1997. 'Women, Resistance and Care: An Ethnographic Study of Nursing Auxiliary Work', *Work Employment and Society* 11(1): 47–63.

Lee, S. et al. 2006. 'Stigmatizing Experience and Structural Discrimination Associated with the Treatment of Schizophrenia in Hong Kong', *Social Science and Medicine* 62(7), 1685–96.

Leibing, A. 2002. 'Flexible Hips? On Alzheimer's Disease and Aging in Brazil', *Journal of Cross-Cultural Gerontology* 17(3): 213–32.

―――― 2006. *Divided Gazes: Alzheimer's Disease, the Person Within, and Death in Life*. New Brunswick: Rutgers University Press.
Leslie, C.M. 1969. 'Modern India's Ancient Medicine', *Society* 6(8): 46–55.
―――― 1976. 'The Ambiguities of Medical Revivalism in Modern India', in C.M. Leslie (ed.), *Asian Medical Systems: A Comparative Study*. Berkeley: University of California Press, pp. 356–67.
―――― 1989. 'Indigenous Pharmaceuticals, the Capitalist World System, and Civilization', *Kroeber Anthropological Society Papers* 69-70: 23–31.
Li, S. and J.L. Chou. 1997. 'Communication with the Cancer Patient in China', *Annals of The New York Academy of Sciences* 809: 243–48.
Liechty, M. 2005. 'Carnal Economies: The Commodification of Food and Sex in Kathmandu', *Cultural Anthropology* 20(1): 1–38.
Lilly USA LLC. 2009. 'Zyprexa® (olanzapine) Prescribing Information'. http://pi.lilly.com/us/zyprexa-pi.pdf, accessed on 30 July 2009.
Linden, M. et al. 1999. 'The Prescribing of Psychotropic Drugs by Primary Care Physicians: An International Collaborative Study', *Journal of Clinical Psychopharmacology* 19(2): 132–40.
Lindstrom, H.A. et al. 2006. 'Medication Use to Treat Memory Loss in Dementia: Perspectives of Persons with Dementia and their Caregivers', *Dementia* 5(1): 27–50.
Link, B.G. and J.C. Phelan. 2001. 'Conceptualizing Stigma', *Annual Review of Sociology* 27(1): 363–85.
Long, S.O. 2004. 'Cultural Scripts for a Good Death in Japan and the United States: Similarities and Differences', *Social Science and Medicine* 58(5): 913–28.
Luce, E. 2006. *In Spite of the Gods: The Strange Rise of Modern India*. London: Little Brown.
Luppa, M. et al. 2008. 'Prediction of Institutionalisation in Dementia', *Dementia and Geriatric Cognitive Disorders* 26(1): 65–78.
Lynch, K. and E. McLaughlin. 1995. 'Caring Labour and Love Labour', in P. Clancy et al. (eds), *Irish Society: Sociological Perspectives*. Dublin: Institute of Public Administration, pp. 250–92.
Madan, T.N. 2004. *India's Religions: Perspectives from Sociology and History*. New Delhi: Oxford University Press.
Mahajan, S. 2006. 'Problems of Urban Senior Citizens in India', *Indian Journal of Social Research* 47(1): 63–73.
Malhotra, S. et al. 2001. 'Drug Related Medical Emergencies in the Elderly: Role of Adverse Drug Reactions and Non-Compliance', *Postgraduate Medical Journal* 77(913): 703–07.
Malik, I. and A. Qureshi. 1997. 'Communication with Cancer Patients: Experiences in Pakistan', *Annals of the New York Academy of Sciences* 809: 300–08.
Manderson, L. 1986. *Shared Wealth and Symbol: Food, Culture and Society in Oceania and Southeast Asia*. Cambridge: Cambridge University Press.
―――― 1996. *Sickness and the State: Health and Illness in Colonial Malaya, 1870-1940*. Cambridge: Cambridge University Press.
Marcus, E.L. and E.M. Berry. 1998. 'Refusal to Eat in the Elderly', *Nutrition Reviews* 56(6): 163–71.

Marcus, G.E. 1995. 'Ethnography In/Of the World System: The Emergence of Multi-Sited Ethnography', *Annual Review of Anthropology* 24: 95–117.
Markovic, M. 2006. 'Analyzing Qualitative Data: Health Care Experiences of Women with Gynecological Cancer', *Field Methods* 18(4): 413–29.
Marriott, M. 1976. 'Hindu Transactions: Diversity Without Dualisms', in B. Kapferer (ed.), *Transaction and Meaning: Directions in the Anthropology of Exchange and Symbolic Behavior*. Philadelphia: Institute for the Study of Human Issues, pp. 109–42.
Marshall, P.A. 2006. 'Informed Consent in International Health Research', *Journal of Empirical Research on Human Research Ethics* 1(1): 25–42.
Martyres, R.F., D. Clode and J.M. Burns. 2004. 'Seeking Drugs or Seeking Help? Escalating "Doctor Shopping" by Young Heroin Users before Fatal Overdose', *Medical Journal of Australia* 180(5): 211–14.
Mathuranath, P.S. et al. 2005. 'Instrumental Activities of Daily Living Scale for Dementia Screening in Elderly People', *International Psychogeriatrics* 17(3): 461–74.
Mattingly, C. 1994. 'The Concept of Therapeutic "Emplotment"', *Social Science and Medicine* 38(6): 811–22.
Mauss, M. 1923, 1990. *The Gift: Forms and Functions of Exchange in Archaic Societies*. London: Routledge.
McCabe, L.F. 2006. 'The Cultural and Political Context of the Lives of People with Dementia in Kerala, India', *Dementia* 5(1): 117–36.
McDonald, K., M. Bartos and D. Rosenthal. 2001. 'Australian Women Living with HIV/AIDS are More Sceptical than Men about Antiretroviral Treatment', *AIDS Care: Psychological and Socio-medical Aspects of AIDS/HIV* 13(1): 15–26.
McLean, A. 2007. *The Person in Dementia: A Study of Nursing Home Care in the US*. Orchard Park: Broadview Press.
McLean, A. and A. Leibing. 2007. *The Shadow Side of Fieldwork: Exploring the Blurred Borders between Ethnography and Life*. Oxford: Blackwell.
Medical Council of India. 2012. Annual Report 2011–2012. http://www.mciindia.org/pdf/Annual%20Report.pdf, accessed on 16 December 2013.
Mehrotra, N. and S. Vaidya. 2008. 'Exploring Constructs of Intellectual Disability and Personhood in Haryana and Delhi', *Indian Journal of Gender Studies* 15(2): 317–40.
Merleau-Ponty, M. 2007. 'The Phenomenology of Perception', in M. Lock and J. Farquhar (eds), *Beyond the Body Proper: Reading the Anthropology of Material Life*. Durham: Duke University Press, pp. 133–49.
Miller, W.I. 1997. *The Anatomy of Disgust*. Cambridge: Harvard University Press.
Mines, D.P. 1989. 'Hindu Periods of Death "Impurity"', *Contributions to Indian Sociology* 23(1): 103–30.
Mintz, S.W. 1985. *Sweetness and Power: The Place of Sugar in Modern History*. New York: Viking.
―――― 1996. 'Food and its Relationship to Concepts of Power', in S.W. Mintz (ed.), *Tasting Food, Tasting Freedom: Excursions into Eating, Culture, and the Past*. Boston: Beacon Press, pp. 17–32.

Moe, K.S. 2003. *Women, Family, and Work: Writings in the Economics of Gender*. Oxford: Blackwell.
Mol, A. 2008. *The Logic of Care: Health and the Problem of Patient Choice*. London: Routledge.
Mooij, J. 1999. 'Food Policy in India: The Importance of Electoral Politics in Policy Implementation', *Journal of International Development* 11(4): 625–36.
Moreira, T. and P. Palladino. 2005. 'Between Truth and Hope: On Parkinson's Disease, Neurotransplantation and the Production of the "Self"', *History of the Human Sciences* 18(3): 55–82.
Mukhophadhyay, A. 1989. 'Public Health Services in a Mess', *Economic and Political Weekly* 24(31): 1751.
Mullan, F. 2006. 'Doctors for the World: Indian Physician Emigration', *Health Affairs* 25(2): 380–93.
Murthy, A.K.S. and R.L. Parker. 1973. 'New Methods for Assessing Healthcare Delivery System', *Indian Journal of Medical Education* 12(3/4): 269–77.
Nandy, A. 1995. *The Savage Freud and Other Essays on Possible and Retrievable Selves*. Princeton: Princeton University Press.
Narayan, U. 1997. *Dislocating Cultures: Identities, Traditions, and Third-World Feminism*. New York: Routledge.
National Human Rights Commission of India. 1999. *Quality Assurance in Mental Health*. New Delhi.
National Capital Region Planning Board. 2010. *Regional Plan 2021*. New Delhi: Ministry of Urban Development, Government of India.
Navarro, V. 1976. *Medicine Under Capitalism*. New York: Prodist.
_____ 1978. *Class Struggle, the State, and Medicine: An Historical and Contemporary Analysis of the Medical Sector in Great Britain*. London: Robertson.
_____ 1982. *Imperialism, Health and Medicine*. London: Pluto.
_____ 1988. 'Professional Dominance or Proletarianization?: Neither', *Milbank Quarterly* 66 (Supplement 2): 57–75.
National Crime Records Bureau (NCRB). 2008. 'Snapshots 2008'. Delhi.
Netscribes. 2009. 'Pharmacy Retail Market in India'. http://rxsupport.webs.com/Market%20picture.pdf, accessed on 17 December 2013.
Nichter, M. 1986. 'The Primary Health Center as a Social System: PHC, Social Status, and the Issue of Team-Work in South Asia', *Social Science and Medicine* 23(4): 347–55.
_____ 1996a. 'Paying For What Ails You: Sociocultural Issues Influencing the Ways and Means of Therapy Payment in South India', in M. Nichter and M. Nichter (eds), *Anthropology and International Health: Asian Case Studies*, 2nd edn. Amsterdam: Gordon and Breach, pp. 239–64.
_____ 1996b. 'Pharmacueticals and the Commodification of Health', in M. Nichter and M. Nichter (eds), *Anthropology and International Health: Asian Case Studies* 2nd edn. Amsterdam: Gordon and Breach, pp. 265–326.
_____ 2008. 'Coming to Our Senses: Appreciating the Sensorial in Medical Anthropology', *Transcultural Psychiatry* 45(2): 163–97.

Nichter, M. and J.J. Thompson. 2006. 'For My Wellness, Not Just My Illness: North Americans' Use of Dietary Supplements', *Culture Medicine and Psychiatry* 30(2): 175–222.
Nichter, M. and D. Van Sickle. 2002. 'The Challenges of India's Health and Healthcare Transition', in A. Ayres and P. Oldenburg (eds), *India Briefing: Quickening the Pace of Change*. Armonk: Asia Society, pp. 159–96.
Nichter, M. and N. Vuckovic. 1994. 'Agenda for an Anthropology of Pharmaceutical Practice', *Social Science and Medicine* 39(11): 1509–25.
Nolan, M.R. et al. 2004. 'Beyond Person-Centred Care: A New Vision for Gerontological Nursing', *Journal of Clinical Nursing* 13(3a): 45–53.
Nussbaum, M.C. 2004. *Hiding from Humanity: Disgust, Shame, and the Law*. Princeton: Princeton University Press.
Oldani, M.J. 2004. 'Thick Prescriptions: Toward an Interpretation of Pharmaceutical Sales Practices', *Medical Anthropology Quarterly* 18(3): 325–56.
Olszewski, B., D. Macey and L. Lindstrom. 2006. 'The Practical Work of Coding: An Ethnomethodological Inquiry', *Human Studies* 29(3): 363–80.
Orenstein, H. 1970. 'Death and Kinship in Hinduism: Structural and Functional Interpretations', *American Anthropologist* 72(6): 1357–77.
Ory, M.G. et al.1999. 'Prevalence and Impact of Caregiving: A Detailed Comparison Between Dementia and Nondementia Caregivers', *The Gerontologist* 39(2): 177–86.
Osuri, G. 2008. 'Ash-coloured Whiteness: The Transfiguration of Aishwarya Rai', *South Asian Popular Culture* 6(2): 109–23.
Parkar, S.R., J. Fernandes and M.G. Weiss. 2003. 'Contextualizing Mental Health: Gendered Experiences in a Mumbai Slum', *Anthropology and Medicine* 10(3): 291–308.
Parker, R. and P. Aggleton. 2003. 'HIV and AIDS-related Stigma and Discrimination: A Conceptual Framework and Implications for Action', *Social Science and Medicine* 57(1): 13–24.
Parry, J. 1981. 'Death and Cosmogony in Kashi', *Contributions to Indian Sociology* 15(1/2): 337–65.
_____ 1985. 'Death and Digestion: The Symbolism of Food and Eating in North Indian Mortuary Rites', *Man* 20(4): 612–30.
Patel, V. et al. 1998. 'Poverty, Psychological Disorder and Disability in Primary Care Attenders in Goa, India', *British Journal of Psychiatry* 172(6): 533–36.
_____ 2005. 'Irrational Drug Use in India: A Prescription Survey from Goa', *Journal of Postgraduate Medicine* 51(1): 9–12.
Patel, V. and M. Prince. 2001. 'Ageing and Mental Health in a Developing Country: Who Cares? Qualitative Studies from Goa, India', *Psychological Medicine* 31(1): 29–38.
Patel, V. and M. Varghese. 2004. 'NGOs and Mental Health: Search for Synergy', in S.P. Agarwal (ed.), *Mental Health: An Indian Perspective 1946-2003*. New Delhi: Ministry of Health and Family Services, pp. 145–51.
Patnaik, A. 2009. 'Crime in Delhi'. New Delhi: Delhi Police.
Patterson, T.J. 1987. 'Indian and European Pracitioners of Medicine from the Sixteenth Century', in G.J. Meulenbeld and D. Wujastyk (eds), *Studies on Indian Medical History*. Groningen: Egbert Forsten, pp. 119–30.

Paveza, G.J. et al. 1992. 'Severe Family Violence and Alzheimer's Disease: Prevalence and Risk Factors', *The Gerontologist* 32(4): 493–97.

Peake, S., L. Manderson and H. Potts. 1999. '"Part and Parcel of Being a Woman": Female Urinary Incontinence and Constructions of Control', *Medical Anthropology Quarterly* 13(3): 267–85.

Pereira, B. et al. 2007. 'The Explanatory Models of Depression in Low Income Countries: Listening to Women in India', *Journal of Affective Disorders* 102(1/3): 209–18.

Peters, D.H. 2002. 'Better Health Systems for India's Poor: Findings, Analysis, and Options'. Washington DC: World Bank.

Peters, D.H. and V.R. Muraleedharan. 2008. 'Regulating India's Health Services: To What End? What Future?', *Social Science and Medicine* 66(10): 2133–44.

Pfleiderer, B. 1988. 'The Semiotics of Ritual Healing in a North Indian Muslim Shrine', *Social Science and Medicine* 27(5): 417–24.

'Pharmacy retailing to grow exponentially if FDI norms eased'. 2009. Livemint.com and *Wall Street Journal*. http://www.livemint.com/2009/08/16142344/Pharmacy-retailing-to-grow-exp.html, accessed on 20 December 2013.

Pink, S. 2009. *Doing Sensory Ethnography*. London: SAGE Publications.

Pinto, S. 2004. 'Development without Institutions: Ersatz Medicine and the Politics of Everyday Life in Rural North India', *Cultural Anthropology* 19(3): 337–64.

_____ 2009. 'Crises of Commitment: Ethics of Intimacy, Kin, and Confinement in Global Psychiatry', *Medical Anthropology* 28(1): 1–10.

_____ 2011. 'Rational Love, Relational Medicine: Psychiatry and the Accumulation of Precarious Kinship', *Culture Medicine Psychiatry* 35(3): 376–95.

Polanyi, K. 1957. 'The Economy as Instituted Process', in K. Polanyi, C. Arensberg and H. Pearson (eds), *Trade and Market in the Early Empires: Economies in History and Theory*. New York: Free Press, pp. 243–70.

Polgreen, L. 2010. 'Indian Who Built Yoga Empire Works on Politics.' *The New York Times*. http://www.nytimes.com/2010/04/19/world/asia/19swami.html?_r=0, accessed on 20 December 2013.

Porter, R. 1997. *The Greatest Benefit to Mankind: Medical History of Humanity from Antiquity to the Present*. London: Harper Collins.

_____ 2002. *Blood and Guts: A Short History of Medicine*. London: Allen Lane.

Pound, P. et al. 2005. 'Resisting Medicines: A Synthesis of Qualitative Studies of Medicine Taking', *Social Science and Medicine* 61(1): 133–55.

Prakash, I.J. 1999. *Ageing in India*. Geneva: World Health Organization.

Prince, M. et al. 2004. 'Alzheimer Disease International's 10/66 Dementia Research Group – One Model for Action Research in Developing Countries', *International Journal of Geriatric Psychiatry* 19(2): 178–81.

Prince, M., G. Livingston and C. Katona. 2007. 'Mental Health Care for the Elderly in Low-Income Countries: A Health Systems Approach', *World Psychiatry* 6(1): 5–13.

Prince, M. and P. Trebilco. 2005. 'Mental Health Services for Older People: A Developing Countries Perspective', in B. Draper, P. Melding and H. Brodaty (eds), *Psychogeriatric Service Delivery*. Oxford: Oxford University Press, pp. 33–54.

Procida, M. 2003. 'Feeding the Imperial Appetite: Imperial Knowledge and Anglo-Indian Domesticity', *Journal of Women's History* 15(2): 123–49.

Purohit, B.C. 2001. 'Private Initiatives and Policy Options: Recent Health System Experience in India', *Health Policy and Planning* 16(1): 87–97.
_____ 2004. 'Inter-state Disparities in Health Care and Financial Burden on the Poor in India', *Journal of Health and Social Policy* 18(3): 37–60.
Rabinow, P. 1977. *Reflections on Fieldwork in Morocco*. Berkeley: University of California Press.
Rabinow, P. and W.M. Sullivan. 1987. 'The Interpretive Turn: A Second Look', in P. Rabinow and W.M. Sullivan (eds), *Interpretive Social Science: A Second Look*. Berkeley: University of California Press, pp. 1–30.
Radhakrishna, R. and K. Subbarao. 1997. 'India's Public Distribution System. A National and International Perspective'. Washington DC: World Bank.
Radhakrishnan, R. 2005. 'PE Usha, Hegemonic Masculinities and the Public Domain in Kerala: On the Historical Legacies of the Contemporary', *Inter-Asia Cultural Studies* 6(2): 187–208.
Raguram, R. et al. 2001. 'Cultural Dimensions of Clinical Depression in Bangalore, India', *Anthropology and Medicine* 8(1): 31–46.
Raja, I. 2005. 'Ageing Subjects, Agentic Bodies: Appetite, Modernity and the Middle Class in Two Indian Short Stories in English', *The Journal of Commonwealth Literature* 40(1): 73–89.
Rajagopal, A. 2001. 'Thinking Through Emerging Markets: Brand Logics and Cultural Forms of Political Society in India', *Economic and Political Weekly* 36(9): 773–82.
Ramesh, M., J. Pandit and G. Parthasarathi. 2003. 'Adverse Drug Reactions in a South Indian Hospital: Their Severity and Cost Involved', *Pharmacoepidemiology and Drug Safety* 12(8): 687–92.
Rao, D. 2006. 'Choice of Medicine and Hierarchy of Resort to Different Health Alternatives among Asian Indian Migrants in a Metropolitan City in the USA', *Ethnicity and Health* 11(2): 153–67.
Rao, V.A. 1993. 'Psychiatry of Old Age in India', *International Review of Psychiatry* 5(2/3), 165–70.
Ray, R. and S. Qayum. 2009. *Cultures of Servitude: Modernity, Domesticity, and Class in India*. Stanford: Stanford University Press.
Reddy, V. 2006. 'The Nationalization of the Global Indian Woman', *South Asian Popular Culture* 4(1): 61–85.
Reidpath, D.D., B. Brijnath and K.Y. Chan. 2005. 'An Asia Pacific Six-country Study on HIV-related Discrimination: Introduction', *AIDS Care* 17(Supplement 2): S117–27.
Rhodes, P. et al. 2008. 'The Use of Biomedicine, Complementary and Alternative Medicine, and Ethnomedicine for the Treatment of Epilepsy among People of South Asian Origin in the UK', *BMC Complementary and Alternative Medicine* 8(1): 7.
Rockwood, K., J.E. Graham and S. Fay. 2002. 'Goal Setting and Attainment in Alzheimer's Disease Patients Treated with Donepezil', *Journal of Neurology, Neurosurgery and Psychiatry* 73(5): 500–07.
Rodriguez, J.J.L. et al. 2008. Prevalence of Dementia in Latin America, India, and China: A Population-based Cross-sectional Survey. *The Lancet* 372(9637): 464–74.
Rose, N. 2001. 'The Politics of Life Itself', *Theory Culture Society* 18(6): 1–30.

Rosenthal, P.J. 2001. *Antimalarial Chemotherapy: Mechanisms of Action, Resistance, and New Directions in Drug Discovery*. Totowa: Humana Press.

Routasalo, P.E. et al. 2006. 'Social Contacts and their Relationship to Loneliness among Aged People: A Population-based Study', *Gerontology* 52(3): 181–87.

Roy, A. 1997. *The God of Small Things*. New York: Random House.

Ryan, G.W. and H.R. Bernard. 2003. 'Techniques to Identify Themes', *Field Methods* 15(1): 85–109.

Sainath, P. 2007. 'Farm Suicides in India, the Result of Profit Driven "Free Market" Reforms'. Montreal: Centre for Research on Globalization.

———2013. 'Nearly 2 lakh farm suicides since 1997', *India Together*. http://www.indiatogether.org/2010/jan/psa-suicides.htm, accessed on 18 December 2013.

Salerno, R.A. 2003. *Landscapes of Abandonment: Capitalism, Modernity, and Estrangement*. Albany: State University of New York Press.

Saravanan, B. et al. 2007. 'Belief Models in First Episode Schizophrenia in South India', *Social Psychiatry and Psychiatric Epidemiology* 42(6): 446–51.

——— 2008. 'Perceptions about Psychosis and Psychiatric Services: A Qualitative Study from Vellore, India', *Social Psychiatry and Psychiatric Epidemiology* 43(3): 231–38.

Sarkar, P.K. 2004. 'A Rational Drug Policy', *Indian Journal of Medical Ethics* 1(1): 11–12.

Sato, T. et al. 1995. 'Doctor-shopping Patients and Users of Alternative Medicine among Japanese Primary-care Patients', *General Hospital Psychiatry* 17(2): 115–25.

Savla, J. et al. 2008. 'Home Help Services in Sweden: Responsiveness to Changing Demographics and Needs', *European Journal of Ageing* 5(1): 47–55.

Scharf, T., C. Phillipson, and A.E. Smith. 2005. 'Social Exclusion of Older People in Deprived Urban Communities of England', *European Journal of Ageing* 2(2): 76–87.

Scheltens, P. and E.S. Korf. 2000. 'Contribution of Neuroimaging in the Diagnosis of Alzheimer's Disease and Other Dementias', *Current Opinions in Neurology* 13(4): 391–96.

Schmalz, M.N. 1999. 'Images of the Body in the Life and Death of a North Indian Catholic Catechist', *History of Religions* 39(2): 177–201.

Schulz, R. and L.M. Martire. 2004. 'Family Caregiving of Persons With Dementia: Prevalence, Health Effects, and Support Strategies', *American Journal of Geriatric Psychiatry* 12(3): 240–49.

Schumacher, K.L. et al. 2000. 'Family Caregiving Skill: Development of the Concept', *Research in Nursing and Health* 23(3): 191–203.

Scull, A.T. 1993. *The Most Solitary of Afflictions: Madness and Society in Britain, 1700–1900*. New Haven: Yale University Press.

Sen, A.K. 1981. *Poverty and Famines: An Essay on Entitlement and Deprivation*. Oxford: Oxford University Press.

Seth, R.K. 1973. 'O.R. in Healthcare Delivery – Rural Health Training Centre, Najafgarh', *Indian Journal of Medical Education* 12(3/4): 256–63.

Shah, G., R. Veedon and S. Vasi. 1995. 'Elder Abuse in India', in J.I. Kosberg and J.L. Garcia (eds), *Elder Abuse: International and Cross-cultural Perspectives*. New York: Haworth Press, pp. 101–18.

Shaji, K. et al. 2002. 'Revealing a Hidden Problem: An Evaluation of a Community Dementia Case-finding Program from the Indian 10/66 Dementia Research Network', *International Journal of Geriatric Psychiatry* 17(3): 222–25.

―――― 2003. 'Caregivers of People with Alzheimer's Disease: A Qualitative Study from the Indian 10/66 Dementia Research Network', *International Journal of Geriatric Psychiatry* 18(1): 1–6.

Shaji, S., S. Bose and A. Verghese. 2005. 'Prevalence of Dementia in an Urban Population in Kerala, India', *British Journal of Psychiatry* 186(2): 136–40.

Sharma, O.P. and C. Haub. 2007. 'Is Delhi India's Largest City?' http://www.prb.org/Articles/2007/delhi.aspx, accessed on 1 April 2010.

Shorter, E. 1997. *A History of Psychiatry: From the Era of the Asylum to the Age of Prozac*. New York: John Wiley and Sons.

Singh, K. 1989. *Delhi: A Novel*. Delhi: Penguin.

Sivaramakrishnan, K. 2006. *Old Potions, New Bottles: Recasting Indigenious Medicine in Colonial Punjab (1850-1945)*. New Delhi: Orient Longman.

Small, J.A. et al. 1998. 'The Discourse of Self in Dementia', *Ageing and Society* 18(3): 291–316.

Small, N. et al. 2005. 'Evidence of Cultural Hybridity in Responses to Epilepsy amongst Pakistani Muslims Living in the UK', *Chronic Illness* 1(2): 165–77.

Smith, B.K. 1990. 'Eaters, Food, and Social Hierarchy in Ancient India', *Journal of the American Academy of Religion* 58(2): 177–206.

Sokolovsky, J. 2009a. 'Aging Proletariats in a Twenty-First-Century Indigenous Mexican Community', in J. Sokolovsky (ed.), *The Cultural Context of Aging: Worldwide Perspectives*, 3rd edn. Westport: Praeger, pp. 216–39.

―――― 2009b. 'Aging, Globalization and Societal Transformation', in J. Sokolovsky (ed.), *The Cultural Context of Aging: Worldwide Perspectives*, 3rd edn. Westport: Praeger, pp. 175–83.

Soofi, M.A. 2008. 'Crass is the City', *The Delhi Walla*, 21 June. http://thedelhiwalla.blogspot.com/2008/06/special-crass-is-city.html, accessed on 24 March 2009.

Sorensen, L. et al. 2005. 'Medication Management at Home: Medication-related Risk Factors Associated with Poor Health Outcomes', *Age and Ageing* 34(6): 626–32.

Spielmans, G.I. 2009. 'The Promotion of Olanzapine in Primary Care: An Examination of Internal Industry Documents', *Social Science and Medicine* 69(1): 14–20.

Srinivas, L. 1995. 'Master-Servant Relationship in a Cross-cultural Perspective', *Economic and Political Weekly* 30(5): 269–78.

Srinivas, T. 2006. '"As Mother Made It": The Cosmopolitan Indian Family, "Authentic" Food and the Construction of Cultural Utopia', *International Journal of Sociology of the Family* 32(2): 191–221.

―――― 2007. 'Everyday Exotic: Transnational Spaces, Identity and Contemporary Foodways in Bangalore City', *Food, Culture and Society* 10(1): 85–107.

Srinivasan, S. 2004. 'A Network for the Rational and Ethical Use of Drugs', *Indian Journal of Medical Ethics* 1(1): 13–14.

Steiner, F. 1956. *Taboo*. New York: Philosophical Library Inc.

Streeten, P. 1997. 'Nongovernmental Organizations and Development', *Annals of the American Academy of Political and Social Science* 554: 193–210.

Stromberg, P., M. Nichter and M. Nichter. 2007. 'Taking Play Seriously: Low-level Smoking among College Students', *Culture, Medicine and Psychiatry* 31(1): 1–24.

Surbone, A. 1997. 'Truth-telling, Risk, and Hope', *Annals of the New York Academy of Sciences* 809: 72–79.

Swain, J., B. Heyman and M. Gillman. 1998. 'Public Research, Private Concerns: Ethical Issues in the Use of Open-ended Interviews with People who have Learning Difficulties', *Disability and Society* 13(1): 21–36.

Tandon, M., S. Prabhakar and P. Pandhi. 2002. 'Pattern of Use of Complementary/Alternative Medicine (CAM) in Epileptic Patients in a Tertiary Care Hospital in India', *Pharmacoepidemiology and Drug Safety* 11(6): 457–63.

Taylor, J.S. 2008. 'On Recognition, Caring, and Dementia', *Medical Anthropology Quarterly* 22(4): 313–35.

Thapan, M. 2000. 'The Body in the Mirror: Women and Representation in Contemporary India', in R. Kumar and N. Chandhoke (eds), *Mapping Histories: Essays Presented to Ravinder Kumar*. New Delhi: Tulika, pp. 337–64.

―――― 2001. 'Adolescence, Embodiment and Gender Identity in Contemporary India: Elite Women in a Changing Society', *Women's Studies International Forum* 24(3/4): 359–71.

Thara, R., R. Padmavati and T.N. Srinivasan. 2004. 'Focus on Psychiatry in India', *British Journal of Psychiatry* 184(4): 366–73.

The 10/66 Dementia Research Group. 2004. 'Care Arrangements for People with Dementia in Developing Countries', *International Journal of Geriatric Psychiatry* 19(2): 170–77.

Tillmann-Healy, L.M. 2003. 'Friendship as Method', *Qualitative Inquiry* 9(5): 729–49.

Townsend, J., M. Godfrey and T. Denby. 2006. 'Heroines, Villains and Victims: Older People's Perceptions of Others', *Ageing and Society* 26(6): 883–900.

Traphagan, J.W. 1998. 'Localizing Senility: Illness and Agency among Older Japanese', *Journal of Cross-Cultural Gerontology* 13(1): 81–98.

―――― 2009. 'Brain Failure, Late Life and Culture in Japan', in J. Sokolovsky (ed.), *The Cultural Context of Aging: Worldwide Perspectives*, 3rd edn. Westport: Praeger, pp. 568–75.

Trawick, M. 1990a. 'The Ideology of Love in a Tamil Family', in O.M. Lynch (ed.), *Divine Passions: The Social Construction of Emotion in India*. Berkeley: University of California Press, pp. 37–64.

―――― 1990b. *Notes on Love in a Tamil Family*. Berkeley: University of California Press.

―――― 1995. 'Writing the Body and Ruling the Land: Western Reflections on Chinese and Indian Medicine', in D.G. Bates (ed.), *Knowledge and the Scholarly Medical Traditions*. Cambridge: Cambridge University Press, pp. 279–96.

Trivedi, A. 2003. 'Knowledge, Awareness and Attitude Regarding Dementia in India', *International Psychogeriatrics* 15 (Supplement 2): 320.

Twigg, J. 2000. 'Carework as a Form of Bodywork', *Ageing and Society* 20(4): 389–411.

Uberoi, P. 1998. 'The Diaspora Comes Home: Disciplining Desire in DDLJ', *Contributions to Indian Sociology* 32(2): 305–36.

UNICEF. 2009. 'Children's Issues – Nutrition'. http://www.unicef.org/india/children_2356.htm, accessed on 26 November 2009.

USAID. 2008. 'Private Health Insurance in India: Promise and Reality'. Washington DC.
Van der Geest, S. and S.R. Whyte. 1988. *The Context of Medicines in Developing Countries: Studies in Pharmaceutical Anthropology*. Dordrecht: Kluwer Academic Publishers.
Van der Veer, P. 1989. 'The Power of Detachment: Disciplines of Body and Mind in the Ramanandi Order', *American Ethnologist* 16(3): 458–70.
Van Hollen, C. 2003. 'Invoking Vali: Painful Technologies of Modern Birth in South India', *Medical Anthropology Quarterly* 17(1): 49–77.
Van Wessel, M. 2004. 'Talking about Consumption: How an Indian Middle Class Dissociates from Middle Class Life', *Cultural Dynamics* 16(1): 93–116.
Van Willigen, J., and Chadha, N.K. 1999. *Social Aging in a Delhi Neighborhood*. Westport: Bergin and Garvey.
Vanderpool, H.Y. and G.B. Weiss. 1987. 'Ethics and Cancer: A Survey of the Literature', *Southern Medical Journal* 80(4): 500–506.
Varghese, M. and V. Patel. 2004. 'The Greying of India: Mental Health Perspective', in S. P. Agarwal (ed.), *Mental Health: An Indian Perspective 1946-2003*. New Delhi: Ministry of Health and Family Services, pp. 240–48.
Varma, P. 1998. *Great Indian Middle Class*. New Delhi: Viking.
Vas, C.J. et al. 2001. 'Prevalence of Dementia in an Urban Indian Population', *International Psychogeriatrics* 13(4): 439–50.
Vatuk, S. 1969. 'Reference, Address, and Fictive Kinship in Urban North India', *Ethnology*, 8(3): 255–72.
———— 1990. '"To Be A Burden On Others": Dependency Anxiety among the Elderly in India', in O.M. Lynch (ed.), *Divine Passions: The Social Construction of Emotion in India*. Berkeley: University of California Press, pp. 64–88.
Vibha, P., S. Saddichha and R. Kumar. 2008. 'Attitudes of Ward Attendants towards Mental Illness: Comparisons and Predictors', *International Journal of Social Psychiatry* 54(5): 469–78.
Victor, C. et al. 2000. 'Being Alone in Later Life: Loneliness, Social Isolation and Living Alone', *Reviews in Clinical Gerontology* 10(4): 407–17.
Vidal, D., E. Tarlo and V. Dupont. 2000. 'The Alchemy of an Unloved City', in V. Dupont, E. Tarlo and D. Vidal (eds), *Delhi: Urban Space and Human Destinies*. New Delhi: Manohar Publishers and Distributors, pp. 15–25.
Vitaliano, P.P., J. Zhang and J.M. Scanlan. 2003. 'Is Caregiving Hazardous to One's Physical Health? A Meta-Analysis', *Psychological Bulletin* 129(6): 946–72.
Von Schmädel, D. and B. Hochkirchen. 1987. 'The Results of Analysis Based on a Video of Consultations in Five *Āyurveda* Medical Practices', in G.J. Meulenbeld and D. Wujastyk (eds), *Studies on Indian Medical History*. Groningen: Egbert Forsten, pp. 225–32.
Warren, N. and L. Manderson. 2008. 'Constructing Hope – Dis/continuity and the Narrative Construction of Recovery in the Rehabilitation Unit', *Journal of Contemporary Ethnography* 37(2): 180–201.
Whittemore, R., S.K. Chase and C.L. Mandle. 2001. 'Validity in Qualitative Research', *Qualitative Health Research* 11(4): 522–37.

World Bank. 2013. 'World Development Indicators'. http://data.worldbank.org/indicator/SH.XPD.PUBL/countries, accessed on 17 December 2013.

World Health Organization. 2005. 'India', in *Mental Health Atlas 2005*. Geneva: pp. 232–35.

―――― 2009. 'Rational Use of Medicines'. http://www.who.int/medicines/areas/rational_use/en/, accessed on 4 September 2009.

―――― 2013. 'World Health Statistics 2013'. Geneva: pp. 122.

World Health Organization and the National Institute of Aging. 2011. 'Global Health and Aging'. http://www.who.int/ageing/publications/global_health/en/, accessed on 20 December 2013.

Wimo, A. et al. 2013. 'The Worldwide Economic Impact of Dementia 2010', *Alzheimers and Dementia: The Journal of the Alzheimer's Association* 9(1): 1–11.

Wujastyk, D. 2003. *The Roots of Ayurveda: Selections from Sankskrit Medical Writings*. London: Penguin Books.

Yang, L.H. et al. 2007. 'Culture and Stigma: Adding Moral Experience to Stigma Theory', *Social Science and Medicine* 64(7): 1524–35.

Yang, L.H. and A. Kleinman. 2008. '"Face" and the Embodiment of Stigma in China: The Cases of Schizophrenia and AIDS', *Social Science and Medicine* 67(3): 398–408.

Zhang, H. 2009. 'The New Realities of Aging in Contemporary China: Coping with the Decline in Family Care', in J. Sokolovsky (ed.), *The Cultural Context of Aging: Worldwide Perspectives*, 3rd edn. Westport: Praeger, pp. 196–215.

INDEX

f denotes figures, n denotes notes, t denotes tables

10/66 Dementia Research Group, 14

adakkam (containment) as an aspect of love, 185
Addlakha, R., 125, 126
adimai (servitude) as an aspect of love, 185
advertisement campaigns
　for Alzheimer's awareness, 40
　for *Horlicks*, 122
　for organ donations, 179
aged care facilities
　attitudes towards, 97–98
　refusal to admit dementia patients, 154
ageing
　and dietary expectations, 120–21
　local idioms associated with, 3–4
　modernity and contextual frameworks for, 6–8
　normal social markers of, 5
Aggarwal, K.P. (person with dementia), 44, 94, 141
Aggarwal, Mamta (carer), 49, 78
Aggarwal, Sita (carer), 44, 55, 94–95, 127–28
Aggleton, P., 156
allopathic doctors, 52
　dietary recommendations, 126
　registered practitioners, 77
Al-Razi, Muhammad B. Zakariya, 61
Alzheimer's and Related Disorders Society of India (ARDSI), 14, 20, 32, 88 *See also* ARDSI-DC and ARDSI-Kerala
Alzheimer's and Related Disorders Society of India – Delhi Chapter (ARDSI-DC), 3, 20–22, 35–36

　attendant training, 108–9
　Founders Day, 21, 89
　funding sources, 88–90
　information handbooks, 50
　level of support for families, 35–36
　links with OPDs, 45–46
　make-up of volunteers and members, 21
　recruiting participants through, 20
Alzheimer's and Related Disorders Society of India – Kerala Chapter, 162–63, 164, 166, 169
Alzheimer's disease
　barriers to early diagnosis, 42
　diagnosis delivery methods, 49–51
　difference from *buddhāpan*, 48, 49, 57
Alzheimer's Disease International, 20, 40
Anglophone cultural scripts around death, 175t
annabrahma, 132
anpu See love
antipsychotic medications, 72–73
Anu, Sandra (attendant), 112, 113, 137
apadharma, 132
Appadurai, A., 118, 119, 133
ARDSI *See* Alzheimer's and Related Disorders Society of India (ARDSI)
ARDSI-DC *See* Alzheimer's and Related Disorders Society of India – Delhi Chapter (ARDSI-DC)
ARDSI-DC 'Memory Clinics' *See* Out Patient Departments (OPDs)
Arora, A.P. (person with dementia), 121, 134, 184
Arora, Mrigakshi (carer), 121
Arora, Vandhana (carer), 74, 108, 109–10, 118, 121, 154

arranged marriages, 185
ashramas life stage, 5
Asian cultural scripts around death, 175t
Association of the Dead, 153
Aṣṭāṅgahrdaya (*The Heart of Medicine*), 64
attendants *See* paid attendants
Auliya, Nizamuddin, 37n7
a:ya (maid), 108 *see also* paid attendants
Āyurveda
 ethics and consent within, 64
 historical foundations of, 61–62
 professionalization of, 79
AYUSH, 64

babas, 62, 85n3
bahūs see daughter-in-law
Banerjee, B., 120
Banerji, D., 101–2
Bartlett, R., 159–60
Bates, D., 62, 64
beauty ideals in India, 169
Begum, Jehan Ara, 37n7
Bhagat, Karamjit (person with dementia), 53–54, 132, 165–66
Bhagat, Nina (carer), 2, 45, 52, 53–54, 78, 80, 92, 93, 97, 132, 133–34, 150, 187
Bhagavad-Gita, 62
Bhatia, B.M., 135–36n5
Bhatnagar, Sunil, Dr., 50–51
bhojan, 132
bhuj, 134
bhu:kh, 130
Bhūlnā (memory loss), 3
Bible, 62
biomedical technology, use in diagnostic process, 47–48
biomedicine, 60, 63
 difference from traditional medicine, 64
black magic practitioners *See kala jādū*
blessing, *See pra-ṇām*
boke (senility), 4
Bollywood films, 157–58
 promotion of idealised beauty, 169
Bose, Dr., 45, 137
brahmacharya life stage, 5
brahmanas, 85n2
Briggs, K., 27

buddhāpan, 41, 45, 138
 difference from Alzheimer's, 48, 49, 57
būṛhā, *See buddhāpan*

carers, 2
 administration of medications, 72–76
 breaking point, 96–98
 commemorating deceased family members, 176
 coping mechanisms during late stages of dementia, 172–73
 dealing with incontinence, 127–28
 depression suffered by, 93–94
 emotional and physical costs to, 93
 externalized stigma, 146, 148–49
 funeral choices for deceased, 176
 guilt felt by, 101
 internalized stigma, 145–46
 links between consumption and identities, 189–190
 loneliness felt by, 138, 150–52
 reaction to stigma, 150, 152
 role of spouses in caregiving, 43
 somatic complaints, 95
 suffering felt by, 150–51
 using food to manage symptoms, 126–27
 violence towards person with dementia, 53–55
 widowed, 39–40, 173, 176–77
 See also primary carers; secondary carers
carework, 9–10
 dealing with dirt/pollution in, 127–29
 as moral practice, 9, 190–91
 See also sevā
caste, 24, 117
 barriers, 110
Central Government of India, 46, 156n1
Chanchala (person with dementia), 162–63
Chand, Helen Meena (person with dementia), 74, 75, 160–61, 168, 172, 173, 174
Chand, Shivbaksh (carer), 2, 27, 75, 95, 122–23, 127, 138, 144, 153–54, 173, 175–76, 177, 187
childishness, *See chinnan*

Chinese perceptions of mental function, 3–4
chinnan (childishness), 3
cholinesterase inhibitors, 71, 73
Chopra, Chintu (carer), 48, 118, 125, 133
Chopra, Kundan Lal (carer), 29, 73, 75, 103, 118, 144, 169
Chopra, Meera (person with dementia), 73, 141, 160–61, 168
Chopra, Rubina (carer), 95, 125, 144
class politics
    in doctor-patient relationships, 64, 69–71
    influence in medical interventions, 178
Clean Delhi Drive, 108, 115n7
Cohen, L., 2, 3, 7, 8, 11n4, 95, 120, 144, 172, 191
Coleman, L., 151
Complaints of a Dutiful Daughter (film), 188
consent *See* informed consent
consumption
    and beauty, 168–69
    links to carers' identities, 189–190
    middle-class perspective on, 92–93
containment as an aspect of love, 185, 189
costs, 87–113
    objective, 93, 99, 107
    of care for middle-class families, 90–93
    of care per person, 91t
    of formal and informal care, 87–88
    of institutionalized care, 98–102
    of pharmaceutical industry, 102–7
    in South Asia, 88
    subjective, 87, 93, 100–102, 113–14
critical ethnography, 13
Crocker, J.B., 139
cure *See ilāj*

dargāh, 36, 37n7
Das, J., 178
Das, R., 81
Das, V., 81, 125, 126, 139, 168
data, 32–36
    analysis, 32–33
    limitations of, 33–36
daughter-in-law, 5, 144, 148

Davis, D.H.J., 159–160
Dawar, Garima, 130
death *See* dying process
dekh (to see), 41–56, 141
dekhānā: See dekh
dekhnā: See dekh
Deleuze, G., 140
Delhi
    breakdown of age demographic, 15–16
    lives of upper class and elite, 18–19
    reasons for undertaking work in, 14–15
    Valentine's Day, 183
    wealth and poverty markers, 37n1
dementia
    cross-cultural perspectives on, 3–5
    difference from *buddhāpan*, 48, 49, 57
    early indicators and diagnostic features of, 41–45
    effect on parent-child dynamics, 187–88
    ethics procedures for projects involving, 30, 32
    increase in prevalence of, 2–3, 88
    interviews with families, 27
    local idioms associated with, 3, 6
    modernity frameworks for, 6–8
    pharmaceutical drugs for, 71–76
    social etiologies for, 55–56, 57
    in Western settings, 4
dementia care
    cost benefits of using pharmaceuticals, 107
    cost of care for middle-class families, 90–93
    cost of care per person, 91t
    costs in South Asia, 88
    costs of, 87–113
    costs of formal and informal care, 87–88
    government health funding, 88–90
    person-centered, 159–160
    short-term respite programmes, 88, 97
    through nursing, sociology and gerontology disciplines, 9
    See also institutionalized care

dementia diagnostic process, 41–57
    diagnosis as result of emotional trauma, 44–45
    diagnosis as result of other medical health conditions, 43–44
    diagnosis delivery methods, 49–51
    early indicators for diagnosis, 41–45
    families' reactions and acceptance of diagnosis, 51–56
    health pathways available, 45–51
    problems with using standard screening methods, 46–47
    in public hospital setting, 46–48 *see also sarkari* hospitals
    relocation and associated problems, 42–43
    use of biomedical technology in, 47–48
dementia participants *See* persons with dementia
Department of *Āyurveda*, Yoga and Naturopathy, *Unani*, Siddha and Homeopathy (AYUSH), 64
dependency anxieties of older people, 6
depression
    in carers, 93–94
    somatic complaint associated with, 95
desi dava:i (local medicine), 68, 85–86n6 *See also* traditional medicine
Desjarlais, R., 162, 163
Dewing, J., 30, 37n6 *See also* Process Consent Method
Dharmashastra, 61, 85n2, 132
Diagnostic and Statistical Manual Version IV (DSM-IV), 41, 51
Diagnostic and Statistical Manual Version V (DSM-V), 57–58n2
dikhnā: see dekh
dirt
    and cleaning, 127–29, 148–49
    in food, 118–19
    typical sensory reactions to, 128
discrimination
    difference from stigma, 139
    institutional, 152–55
disgust response, 128
    links to stigma, 149
dividuals, concepts of, 117–18, 166–67
Divya Yog Mandir Trust, 83

Dixit, Sheila, 16
doctor shopping, 10, 51–53, 57, 59, 76, 84, 103
doctor-patient relationships, 10, 84
    class politics in, 64–65, 69–71
    gifting etiquette, 106–7
    past and present, 64–67
    in *sarkari* hospitals, 66, 104–5
doctors
    attitudes towards dementia patients, 45, 154–55
    factors affecting truth telling practices, 49–51, 65
    shortage of, 4, 68, 101
domestic citizenship, 125–29
domestic economies, 107–13
donepezil, 71
Dossa, P., 125
Douglas, M., 128
Dreze, J., 131
Dumit, J., 49
Dumont, L., 24
dying process
    cross-cultural perspectives on, 174, 175t
    cultural scripts around, 174–77, 181
    funeral rites, 176
    Hindu ideals, 175
    political economies of, 178–81

elder care
    measures of *sevā*, 92
    traditional forms of, 5–6
Eleventh Five Year Plan (2007–2012), 88
elimai (simplicity) as an aspect of love, 185
ethics
    procedures for dementia projects, 30, 32
    formal ethics, 32
    informal ethics, 32
    institutional ethics, 32 personal ethics, 32
ethnographic approaches, 13
    limitations of, 34–35
ethopolitics, 179, 180
'eve-teasing,' 16

exchanges
 attendant-family, 111–13
 doctor-patient, 103–4
exploitation of patients and attendants, 101–2, 112–13

fakirs, 85n3
familial titles, 5
Famine (Sharma), 129 *See also Kāl* (Saraswat)
famines, 131, 135–36n5
Farmer, P., 71
fast track courts, 156n1
fieldwork
 challenges of, 12–13, 159–62
financial security and safeguards, 43
 legislation for protection of, 153–54
folk medicine, *See* transcendental medicine
food
 cooking as act of caring, 122–25
 cultural significance of, 117–19
 dietary expectations of elders, 120–21
 dirt in food preparation, 119
 Hindu philosophies on, 132
 homogenizing effects of, 118–19
 links between identities and, 117–20, 135
 links to sex, 134
 nostalgia for home cooking, 117
 pleasure of sweets and feeding, 133–35
 refusal to eat, 129–133
 See also gastropolitics; *ghar ka kha:na* (home cooking)
Foucault, M., 122
Francis (person with dementia), 164
Francis, Dr (faith healer), 82
Freidson, E., 66

galantamine, 71, 86n9
galenic medicine *See* biomedicine
Gammeltoft, T.M., 125
gastropolitics, 117, 133
Gauri (person with dementia), 168–69
Gerriamma (person with dementia), 65
ghar ka kha:na (home cooking), 116–19
Ghosh, Somya (ARDSI volunteer), 73, 88–89
gifting *see* doctor-patient relationships

The God of Small Things (Roy), 188
Goffman, E., 138
gone sixtyish, 3, 8 *see also saṭhiyānā*
Gopalan, L., 158
government hospitals *See* Out Patient Departments (OPDs); *sarkari* hospitals
Government of India, 32
 fast track courts, 156n1
 health funding, 88–90
 incorporating traditional medicine into national health programmes, 79
 national health programmes, 88
 See also Eleventh Five Year Plan (2007–2012); Twelfth Five Year Plan (2012–2014)
Gowda, Parvati (carer), 42–43, 120, 131, 150, 167
grahasthya life stage, 5
Granado, S., 48
Great Bengal Famine, 131
Great Medical Compendium, 61 *see Kitab al-Djami 'al-kabir*
gurus, 62, 85n3
Guru Ramdev, 82, 83
guṣṣa (aggression), 3

Hahn, H., 47
Ḥakīm, 64, 83
Hamdari, Mr (carer), 24, 54
Hamdari, Mrs (person with dementia), 24, 44, 72–73, 90, 141, 167–68
Hammer, J., 178
hāth-pair (hands and feet), 94–96
healer-patient relationships, 82–84
healthcare systems
 characteristics of, 103
 hierarchies within, 28–29, 101–2, 105–6
The Heart of Medicine, 64
HelpAge India, 125
Hinduism
 philosophy on dying process, 175
 philosophy on food, 63, 131–32
 philosophy on life stages, 5–6
Hoffmann, D., 188
home cooking *See ghar ka kha:na* (home cooking)
homeopathy, 79

home
    as private social spaces, 151–52
    homes as spaces for beauty and consumption, 168–69
Homo Hierarchicus (Dumont), 24
human rights in hospitals, 69–71
hunger *See* starvation and hunger

identities
    employment as source of, 164–65
    feminine, 165
    and food, 117–20
    See also masculinity
ilāj (cure), 59–60
    as driving force in doctor shopping, 76
    etymology of, 61–64
    patients resisting, 75–76
    pharmaceutical, 72f, 103
incontinence, dealing with, 127–28. *See also* dirt
informed consent, 29–31
    in *Āyurvedic* context, 64–65
    cross-cultural differences regarding, 29
institutionalized care
    attitudes towards, 97–98
    costs of, 100–2
    exploitation of patients and attendants in, 101–2
    impact on families, 96–97, 98–102
institutionalized discrimination, 152–55
institution-patient relationships, 69–71
intergenerational living arrangements, 5, 97, 114n4
interviews
    challenges of, 29–30, 160–62
    cross section of families participating in, 23
    with families, 27
    with key service providers (KSPs), 26
    procedures for, 26–27
    transcription process, 32–33
irrational drug use, 102, 104, 114–15n5
Isaacs, P., 34
Isaksen, L., 128
isolation as a result of internalized stigma, 145–46

Jahangir (attendant), 112–13
Jaiswal, Tara (person with dementia), 141, 150
Jaitley, Arvind, 79
Japanese perceptions of mental function and senility, 4
Jeffery, P., 110
Jeffery, R., 110
jhāṛ-poṅćh practitioners, 81
Jones, E., 139

Kakar, S., 134
Káḷ (Saraswat), 129
kala jādū (black magic) practitioners, 62, 81
Kamat, V., 105
Kamini *See* slums
kāmzori (weakness), 94–95, 103, 131
Karan Arjun (film), 157, 158
Kaufman, S., 4, 178
Kaul, Kumud (carer), 24, 142, 187–88
    See also Hamdari, Mrs (person with dementia)
Kaur, Gurneet (carer), 148–49 *See also* Singh, Harinder (person with dementia)
Kaur, Jaspreet (carer), 70, 123, 133, 148–49 *See also* Singh, Harinder (person with dementia)
key service providers (KSPs), 26, 29
Khāmosh (silence), 157
Khan, Inayat, 37n7
Khan, Omar (person with dementia), 38, 43, 53, 81, 89, 131, 146, 173
Khan, Shafia (carer), 38–40, 50, 53, 82, 131, 146, 186
Khare, R., 131, 132
Khusro, Amir, 37n7
kinship and reciprocal relations, 125
    master-servant relationships, 108–13
    terms of address, 5, 17
Kitab al-Djami 'al-kabir (Great Medical Compendium), 61
kitty parties, 21, 37n4
Kitwood, T., 159–60
Kleinman, A., 9, 139, 190
Kochar, Lakshmi Kumari (person with dementia), 121, 168, 172
Kochar, Sarojini (carer), 90, 108
kodumai (cruelty) as an aspect of love, 185
Kontos, P., 9, 160

kshatriyas, 85n2
Kumar, Dr., 66
Kumar, N., 12, 71, 161

Lamb, S., 7, 8, 34, 120, 127, 172, 191
Langford, J., 79
language
    framing chronic diseases in Hindi, 142
    local idioms associated with dementia, 6
    use in diagnosis process, 48–49
Leibing, A., 9, 32
life-stages in Vedic Hindu philosophy, 5
Link, B., 139
local medicine, *See desi dava:i*
local worlds, variability of moral experiences, 140
Lock, M., 139
loneliness, 56, 150–52
Long, S., 174
love
    between carers and spouses, 184–87
    commercialization of, 183
    containment as an aspect of love, 185, 189
    cruelty as an aspect of love, 185
    men, feelings about love, 187
    simplicity as an aspect of love, 185–86
    servitude as an aspect of love, 185–86
    sevā as measure of depth of commitment and love, 186–89
    through anthropological framework, 183–87
    various aspects of, 185
    See also adakkam; adimai; elimai; kodumai; parakkam
low-class families *See* poor families

madness *See pa:gaal*, social signs of
Magnetic Resonance Imaging (MRI), 47–48, 57, 58n3
maids, 108, 150 *see also a:ya* and paid attendants
Maintenance and Welfare of Parents and Senior Citizens Act (2008), 153–54
major neurocognitive disorder, 11n1 *See also* Alzheimer's disease; dementia
Manusmiriti, 85n2
Marriott, M., 117, 166

masculinity
    connections between identity and work, 163–67
    See also men
master-servant relationships, 108–13
Mauss, M., 106
McLean, A., 32
med reps, 104–5
    preference for *sarkari* hospitals, 106
medical dominance, 66, 69–71, 104
medical literature, earliest sources of, 61–62
medical pluralism, 61–63, 77, 83
Mehrotra, N., 125
Mehta, D., 161
memantine, 71
memory and connections to food, 117, 118
memory loss, 3
men
    attitudes towards medication administration, 74–75
    creating meaningful identities, 165–67
    feelings about love, 187
Menon, Radha (carer), 97, 123, 141, 143, 145, 186
Menon, Rajesh (person with dementia), 143, 164, 172
mental health professionals, shortage of, 4, 101
Merleau-Ponty, M., 162
middle-class families, 23
    average wage of, 114n2
    cost of care challenges for, 90–93
    funding help, 90
migration
    impact on familial structures, 6–7
    rural to urban, 15
Miller, W., 128
Mini Mental State Exam (MMSE), 46, 160
Ministry of Health and Family Welfare, 64, 79, 85n1
modernity and dementia, 6–8
Mol, A., 9
Monash University, Human Research Ethics Committee, 32
moral experience, 139–40
Moreira, T., 60
Moses (person with dementia), 164

Mritak Sangh (Association of the Dead), 153–54
Mukherjee, Gautam (person with dementia), 173–74
Mukherjee, Shilpi (carer), 111, 123, 176

Nandy, A., 77
National Capital Region (NCR), 15
National Commission for Senior Citizens, 88
National Institute of Ageing, 88, 190
National Sample Survey Organisation 2004, 37n2
National Trust for the Aged, 88
Navarro, V., 67
nerva frakese (tired brain), 3
neuroimaging, 47–49, 57
NGOS *See* Alzheimer's and Related Disorders Society of India (ARDSI) and its chapters; Alzheimer's and Related Disorders Society of India – Delhi Chapter (ARDSI-DC); HelpAge India
Nichter, M., 48, 105, 107
normal, outwardly presentations
  maintaining 140–42
  risks associated with perceived normalcy, 143–45
nursing perspectives on dementia care, 9
Nussbaum, M., 100
Nvivo software, 32

objective costs of care, 93, 99, 107
observation, 14, 26–27
  in OPDs, 45–46, 104–5
O'Connor, D., 159–60
OPDs *See* Out Patient Departments (OPDs)
organ donations, 178–81
  institutional bureaucracies and impact on, 180–81
  value of, 179
Out Patient Departments (OPDs), 45–46, 104–5
  doctor-patient relationships, 66, 104–5
  numbers of patients treated at, 46

pa:gaal (madness), social signs of, 138, 141–43
paid attendants, 107–13
  difference from servants, 108
  exploitation of, 101–2, 112–13
  families' attitudes towards, 109–10
  physical and emotional stress, 113
  power and agency of, 111–12
  working conditions of, 110–11
palana-posana, 132
Palladino, P., 60
parakkam (habit) as an aspect of love, 185
parent-child relationships and effect of dementia on, 187–88
Parents in India, Children Abroad (PICA), 7
Parker, R., 156
partitioning of India, 23, 37n5
Pather Panchali (film), 120
patients and violation of rights in hospitals, 69–71
person-centered care, 159–60
persons with dementia
  cost of care per person, 91t
  deaths of, 173–74
  difficulties in interviewing, 30–31
  expressions of desire to die, 172–73
  families of, 22–26
  families receiving funding, 90
  information gap and access to health services, 28–29
  love between spouses and, 184
  responses to touch and poetry, 162–63, 167
  stigma, 140–45
  violence towards, 53–55
  work as means of engagement, 163–66
  See also Alzheimer's participants
Pfizer, 105
pharmaceutical drugs, 71
  availability and proliferation of, 102
  for dementia, 71–76
  families' experiences with, 60
  rates of hospitalization from adverse reactions in US and UK, 74
  supervision of dosage levels, 72–76
  types used by dementia patients, 72f
  See also antipsychotic medications
pharmaceutical *ilāj*, 103
pharmaceutical industry
  factors affecting cost of, 102–7
  gifting, 106–7
  worth of, 103
  See also med reps

pharma-economies, 102–7
Phelan, J., 139
Pillai, Nandini (carer), 42, 73, 78, 109, 111, 126–27, 128–29, 154–55
Pinto, S., 48, 110
pīrs, 62, 85n3
Planning Commission of India (2007), 68
pollution *See* dirt
poor families, 23–24, 28
    access to interviews with, 35
Pound, P., 75
pra-ṇām (blessing), 5, 6
Prasad, Hari (person with dementia), 91, 147–48
primary carers
    demographic data of, 25t
    difficulty of categorising, 24, 31
    women as, 55
private health insurance market, 103
private health sector, 67–68
    attitudes towards dementia, 45
    diagnosis delivery methods in, 50–51
private spaces, homes as, 151–52
Process Consent Method, 30–31, 37n6
product executives, *See also* med reps
Protocol to Minimise Interview Distress for People with Dementia, practical applications, 30–31

qawwālī, 36, 37n8
Qu'ran, 62

Rabinow, P., 13
Rai, Aishwarya, 179
Ramdev, Guru, 82, 83
Ranbaxy, 105
Ranjarajan, Meenakshi (person with dementia), 42–43, 120, 167, 168
Al-Razi, Muhammad B. Zakariya, 61
religious healing, *See* transcendental medicine
research designs, 13–14
researcher-participant relations and consent processes, 29–31
Ṛgveda, 61
rivastigmine, 71
Rose, N., 179
Roy, A., 188

Roy, Dr Jacob, 20
rural settings, prevalence rates for dementia, 3

Sadhwani, Suneeta (carer), 2, 24, 50, 56, 91, 94, 95, 118, 137, 138, 147–48 *See also* Prasad, Hari (person with dementia)
sampling strategies, 35–6
Santosh (person with dementia), 164
sanyas life stage, 5, 120
Saraswat, R., 129
sarkari hospitals, 26, 46, 51
    doctor-patient relationships, 66, 104–5
    patients dissatisfaction with, 69
    power hierarchy with patients and families, 69–71
    shortage of doctors, 4, 68
    typical scenario for doctors in, 67–68
Saroj (attendant), 112
Saṭhiyānā (gone sixtyish), 3, 8
secondary carers
    demographic data of, 25t
    difficulty of categorising, 24, 26, 31
selfhood, notions of, 159–160
self-medication practice, 102, 104, 114–15n5
Sen, A., 131
Sen, Nayantara (carer), 2, 24, 44, 52, 54, 69, 72–73, 78, 81–83, 154, 167–68, 187–88 *See also* Hamdari, Mrs (person with dementia)
senility, Japanese perceptions on, 4
sensorial anthroplogy, 13, 135
service *See sevā*
servitude as an aspect of love, 185–86
Sethi, Mrs Chandhana (carer), 27, 59, 60, 74
sevā, 5–6, 41
    as measure of depth of commitment and love, 186–89
    through carework, 94–95, 97, 112, 127–29, 142, 149
    through consumption, 92–93, 189
    through doctor shopping, 52–53, 57
    through food, 10, 121–22, 125, 130
    through kinship, 45, 113
    through medical interventions, 59, 75, 161, 172, 178, 189

sex and sexuality
    links to food, 34, 134
    as taboo subject with interviewees, 34
Sharma, I., 129
Shivanni (homeopath), 79
shudras, 85n2
sight metaphors in dementia, 41–56, 141–45 *See also dekh*
silence, *see Khāmosh*
Singh, Ajit (carer), 70, 148
Singh, Harinder (person with dementia), 70, 74, 148–49
Singh, Josie Dharam (carer), 2, 39–41, 43, 47, 56, 98–102, 109, 114, 133, 144, 150, 172, 176, 178–80, 184
Singh, P.K. (ARDSI-DC volunteer), 137, 138, 178
Singh, Surinder Dharam (person with dementia), 41, 173
single photo emission computed tomography (SPECT) scan, 47
slums
    attendant training for women from, 108–9
    health services in, 35
    impact of gentrification on, 115n7
    working conditions of attendants from, 110–11
social death, 139, 151
social suffering, 139
sociological perspectives on dementia care, 9
Sokolovsky, J., 7
Sood, Namita (carer), 2, 45, 77, 78, 91–92, 110, 174–76, 178–80
SPECT scan, 47
Srinivas, T., 119
Srivastava, Bhageshwari (carer), 78, 108, 111, 118, 141, 150, 154, 188 *See also* Jaiswal, Tara (person with dementia)
starvation and hunger
    politics around, 131–32, 135
    See also bhu:kh; famines
stigma, 10
    defining, 138–140
    difference from discrimination, 139
    internal and external, 145–49, 155–56

links to disgust, 149
opinions on, 137–38
preserving normalcy, 140–42
strategies to dispel, 140–45, 156
Streeten, P., 89–90
stubbornness, *see zid*
subjective costs of care, 87, 93, 100–102, 113–14
suffering felt by carers, 96–100, 150–51
sufi mystics, 37n7
suicide of farmers, 132
Surbone, A., 65

tabeez, 62, 85n4
Talwar, Savitri (carer), 133
Talwar, Sudhansu (person with dementia), 81–82, 133
Tandon, Govind Ballabh (carer), 2, 44, 50, 56, 59, 76, 80, 81, 83–84, 134, 145–46, 152, 187
Tandon, Sheila (person with dementia), 44, 56, 76, 80, 134–35
Taylor, J., 9
test-wallahs, 105–6
Tillmann-Healy, L., 32
tired brain, 3
traditional medicine, 62
    desi dava:i (local medicine), 68, 85–86n6
    dietary recommendations, 126
    difference from biomedicine, 64–65
    overlap with bio- and transcendental medicine, 79
    professionalization of, 77–79
    registered practitioners, 77
    treatments used by families, 76–80
transcendental medicine, 36, 62, 63, 80–84
    blurring of religious boundaries, 83–84
    dietary recommendations, 126
    overlap with bio- and traditional medicine, 79
transcription process, 32–33
Trawick, M., 110, 185
tropical medicine, 63
tube feeding, 129–31
Twelfth Five Year Plan (2012–2014), 88
Tyagi, Inspector, 43, 109, 153

Unani medicine, 61–62
urban settings
  population and cities, 15
  prevalence rates for dementia, 3

Vāgbhata, 64
vaid, 64, 82, 83
Vaidya, S., 125
vaishyas, 85n2
Van Hollen, C., 48
van Wessel, M., 92
vanaprastha life stage, 5, 120
Varma, P., 109
Vatuk, S., 6, 120
Vedas, 61
Vedic Hindusim *See* Hinduism
violence in carers and participants, 53–55

weakness *See kāmzori* (weakness)
wealthy families, 23
  doctor shopping, 52–53
  funding help, 90
WHO, 79

WHO Essential Drugs List, 102
women
  attitudes towards medication administration, 74
  creating meaningful identities, 167–69
  depression in carers, 93–94
  evolving roles, 6–7, 122
  openness about feelings for spouses, 187
  performing *sevā* through cooking, 121–22
  as primary and secondary carers, 24, 55
  somatic complaints, 95
  treatment of women in urban settings, 16–17
World Alzheimer's Day, 21, 89

Yashaswini, Dr., 67–69, 77, 84, 180
yoga therapy, 83
yogaksema, 132

zid (stubbornness), 3